THE LITTLE BOOK OF
PERFUMES

THE LITTLE BOOK OF
PERFUMES

THE HUNDRED CLASSICS

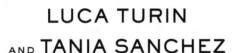

LUCA TURIN
and TANIA SANCHEZ

VIKING

VIKING

Published by the Penguin Group
Penguin Group (USA) Inc., 375 Hudson Street,
New York, New York 10014, U.S.A.
Penguin Group (Canada), 90 Eglinton Avenue East,
Suite 700, Toronto, Ontario, Canada M4P 2Y3
(a division of Pearson Penguin Canada Inc.)
Penguin Books Ltd, 80 Strand, London WC2R 0RL, England
Penguin Ireland, 25 St. Stephen's Green, Dublin 2, Ireland
(a division of Penguin Books Ltd)
Penguin Books Australia Ltd, 250 Camberwell Road, Camberwell,
Victoria 3124, Australia (a division of Pearson Australia Group Pty Ltd)
Penguin Books India Pvt Ltd, 11 Community Centre,
Panchsheel Park, New Delhi–110 017, India
Penguin Group (NZ), 67 Apollo Drive, Rosedale, Auckland 0632,
New Zealand (a division of Pearson New Zealand Ltd)
Penguin Books (South Africa) (Pty) Ltd, 24 Sturdee Avenue,
Rosebank, Johannesburg 2196, South Africa

Penguin Books Ltd, Registered Offices:
80 Strand, London WC2R 0RL, England

First published in 2011 by Viking Penguin,
a member of Penguin Group (USA) Inc.

1 3 5 7 9 10 8 6 4 2

Most of the reviews in this book first appeared in *Perfumes: The Guide*
by Luca Turin and Tania Sanchez (Viking, 2008).

LIBRARY OF CONGRESS CATALOGING IN PUBLICATION DATA
Turin, Luca.
The little book of perfumes : the hundred classics /
Luca Turin and Tania Sanchez.
p. cm.
Includes index.
ISBN 978-0-670-02310-3
1. Perfumes—Miscellanea. I. Sanchez, Tania. II. Title.
TP983.T868 2011
668'.54—dc23   2011026496

Printed in the United States of America
Set in Minion Pro
Designed by Francesca Belanger

For the perfumers

CONTENTS

ACKNOWLEDGMENTS

We would like to give an enormous thank-you to Patricia de Nicolaï, tireless curator of the Osmothèque and the great perfumer behind the Parfums de Nicolaï. Many thanks to all in the perfume industry who helped us this time around, and all the perfume lovers who gave us their support and feedback after the publication of *Perfumes: The A–Z Guide*. Thanks to the good people at the Santa Fe Institute for giving us the perfect place to concentrate on our work, and thanks especially to Janet Rubinstein for enduring all those packages of perfumes. Thanks also to Kathryn Court and all her team at Penguin USA and Peter Carson and all at Profile UK, for proposing this book, and thanks to the marvelous Thomas and Elaine Colchie, terrific agents and even better friends.

AUTHORS' NOTE

Perfume formulas are trade secrets. Short of gas-chromatograph mass spectrometry, it is impossible, for all practical purposes, to get official confirmation that a formula has been changed and how, though it is easy to get rumors off the record. There is plenty of publicly available information on industry restrictions. We judge changes based on what we smell in side-by-side tests of previous years' bottles and new samples, direct from the firms whenever possible.

FOREWORD
by Tania Sanchez

Every buff has a list: the hundred films you must see before dying, the top three cheeseburgers in the northern hemisphere, the ten most overrated paintings, the twenty most idiotic reviews in *Perfumes: The A–Z Guide*, etc. What pleasurable conniptions attend the discovery that someone has ranked *Hellboy II* above *Casablanca* or thinks *Let It Be* trumps *Revolver*! In fact, probably the best reason to make such a list is the easy satisfaction it provides of infuriating so many with so little effort.

The fragrances reviewed in this book are not the greatest of all time—instead, they are those that struck us as far above their peers in quality, inventiveness, or straightforward beauty when we surveyed nearly 1,900 during the writing of *Perfumes: The A–Z Guide*, ignoring all publicity, packaging, and the feelings of friends and neighbors and concentrating solely on the scent. This ruled out fragrances that everyone admires except us, and also fragrances that have suffered at the hands of changing formulas. So even if Tabac Blond at its best deserved, in general opinion, to edge out, say, Badgley Mischka, it was not in any shape to argue for itself at the time, so it's not in.

This slim, rigorously positive volume also eliminates all fragrances we found less than magnificent: good news for readers who believe if you can't say anything nice you shouldn't say anything at all, and bad news for anyone who despises events in which everyone who turns up gets a prize. So if you want to find out what we thought of Paris Hilton's Can Can, you will have to seek the bigger book.

To make up for our arbitrary, ahistorical approach and to satisfy the preference of publishers for multiples of ten, we add, to the ninety-six top-ranked fragrances from our previous book, four brief writings on long-gone fragrances of historical importance. Our impressions are based on reconstructions, from the original formulas, from the Osmothèque, a museum in Versailles devoted to the history of the art of the perfumer. It is not a museum full of pretty crystal, magazine advertisements, and mythologies. It is a place where perfumes sit in cold storage, away from light and abuse, waiting to evaporate up your nose and trigger sensations. We include François Coty's Emeraude, L'Origan, and Chypre, plus a possibly perfect composition by Vincent Roubert, Iris Gris. The first three turn up, in various incarnations, frequently at auctions and estate sales—look for older packaging to avoid cheapened recent versions. The last is almost impossible to find, though one lucky woman we know found a pristine full bottle at a flea market with which she taunts everyone. Aside from such serendipitous finds, watch for demonstrations by the Osmothèque, in Versailles or by their representation in the United States.

The fact that you can no longer buy these scents as they were intended leads us to the irksome issue of changing formulas. Going against my promise to give only good news, I warn you that many of the fragrances we loved, which untold millions have enjoyed for decades, have changed drastically in the last few years because of aggressive regulation on allergens. That is why we have gone to the trouble of adding recent smelling notes on as many fragrances as we could recheck in time.

I confess that I, as a naturally allergic, itchy, and wheezy person, one of these children who had to take a note to the teacher warning against peanuts, who carries an inhaler and fast-acting antihistamines, and who cannot seem to find a shampoo that does not turn her scalp into a dermatological textbook illustration, am very surprised by the industry's ruthless weeding out of allergens in fine fragrance. After all, my allergy is my problem. I would never demand that other people stop wearing red lipstick because I can't, or cease washing their clothes in enzymatic detergents because they could irritate me. Therefore, I find it very surprising that someone has decided I cannot have my L'Heure Bleue ever again because someone else, somewhere, got a red welt. Why can't she wear something else?

This is because every now and then, on a slow news day, an activist group puts out a press release claiming that chemicals found in perfume give you cancer, turn boys into girls, are passed into breast milk, are irritants and sensitizers, and so on. These alarms, often based on effects found at enormous doses, far above amounts you would be exposed to short of falling into a factory vat or drinking the stuff straight, trigger widespread calls to ban perfume. Since perfume is not a toxic, carcinogenic soup and is highly regulated to avoid human or environmental harm, the International Fragrance Association, aka IFRA, needed something to do to prove to the public that they care about health and safety. Therefore, they decided to devote enormous resources to reducing contact dermatitis. And that is why you can't have your old Diorissimo, even if the only reaction you ever had to it was happiness.

Materials used in great quantity were first to fall to bans or restrictions. These include traditionally important ones such as hydroxycitronellal (the only convincing lily-of-the-valley), oakmoss (the bitter, inky forest smell lurking in nearly every classic perfume), birch tar (leather), heliotropin (mimosa), jasmine (jasmine!), eugenol (carnations and mulling spices, adieu), bergamot (the delicious citrus start of Shalimar among many), and others. One of the great ironies of fragrance is that well-meaning activists who fear strange chemicals in perfume have inadvertently encouraged an increase of those chemicals, to replace familiar materials used with no grievous harm for over a hundred years.

For this reason, we did our best to retest fresh, authentic samples of as many of our top-rated perfumes as we could find since 2010 was an important year for compliance in the industry. The results were not all bad, but they weren't all good, either. We note the changes, and if we can't speak for the current version we have noted that too. Some we did not get in time. In other cases, firms were uninterested in marketing any perfume released earlier than five years ago, and some seemed oddly uninterested in their own products at all. However, their indifference may work in your favor: great perfumes without aggressive marketing may be available in their old formulation and old packaging for years in the back stock of perfume shops.

Hunting out old bottles is a pleasurable task, if you are the sort to wander idly through secondhand shops, browse eBay, or stop at every mom-and-pop roadside perfume discounter, with piles of dusty boxes in the back. And if you were to smell every one of these fragrances as they were when they earned our praise, it would be an education as well as an entertainment. They span an enormous range—prim bouquets of white flowers, sour pine-and-sage compositions fit for a desert night, classical milky-musky scents that should waft from fifties mink coats, modern transparent odors that fill the room with traces of herbs or woodsmoke, hairy-chested aromatic things for disco-dancing men with mustaches, Arabian attars of rose and incense, lush and bittersweet balsams for serious ladies, and more, may there always be more. As Luca has said before, perfume is a message in a bottle. While our translations into ordinary speech of what these perfumes say to us in their vaporous language may make interesting reading, in the end we will have done our job only if you seek out these quiet genies lurking in their flasks, release them, give them your full attention, and let them tell you their secrets themselves.

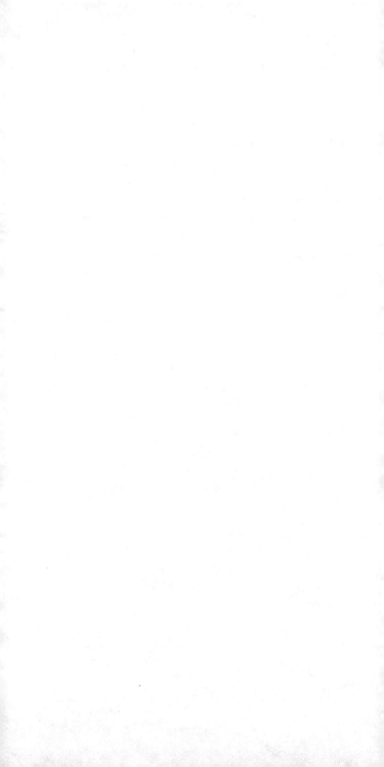

THE LITTLE BOOK OF
PERFUMES

PERFUME REVIEWS

Price
$$$$ OVER $200
$$$ FROM $101 TO $200
$$ FROM $51 to $100
$ FROM $1 to $50

Our indications are based on the standard U.S. retail price of the smallest full-size bottle of the lowest concentration in standard distribution. For example, we will take into account an individually sold one-ounce eau de toilette, but not an eighth-ounce parfum sold only as part of a gift set. We also do not count concentrations below eau de toilette or lotions, soaps, etc. Because sizes, concentrations, and cost of materials vary widely, price indications are intended to help readers shop for fragrances in a given price range and should not be interpreted as a measure of value for money.

31 Rue Cambon (Chanel) *floral ambery* $$$
I cannot remember the last time, if ever, a perfume gave me such an instantaneous impression of ravishing beauty at first sniff. There is an affecting softness, a gentle grace to 31 that beggars belief. Such a classical masterpiece must, by definition, be standing on the shoulders of giants, and identifying them can be a compelling game. At times 31 brings to mind the old Chant d'Arômes, before Guerlain messed with it. There is also a touch of the first Dioressence, that overripe, blowsy milky-fruity note of lactones that Gucci Rush took to its

logical extreme. But Chant d'Arômes was demure, Dior-essence come-hither, and Rush a monochrome. Chanel's 31 does not play games, try to seduce, or attempt to be modern. Perhaps the real precursor of 31 is that flawed masterpiece, Yves Saint Laurent's Champagne. Champagne too was a soft, fruity chypre, but its brassy, plangent treatment of the theme suggested the decadence of a once-great lineage. By contrast, 31 shows that in the higher reaches of art, time is suspended. One of the ten greats of all time, and precious proof that perfumery is not yet dead. LT

In the press pack for 31 Rue Cambon, Chanel boasts of having composed a chypre fragrance without the sine qua non: oakmoss, a resin extracted from a lacy lichen that looks something like frisée and grows mainly on oak trees in Eastern Europe. When cooked into usable form, it becomes a thick goo with a medieval fairy-tale smell of smoke, ink, and forest mulch, which gives the rich and sweet chypre idea its bitter backbone. So what is a chypre without oakmoss? An exercise in illusion via allusion. By arranging a series of familiar cues, 31 Rue Cambon calls to mind other great fragrances, older and recent, and makes you imagine the missing element. That rich iris beginning, substituting a nose-ticklingly dry pepper for the leather, promises Chanel's own Cuir de Russie; floating in and out of focus is the jasmine heart of Diorella, fizzy and bright as cold 7UP; you find a lemon-custard moment that makes you think briefly of Shalimar Light, among others; and oh, that big, singing amber, didn't you meet it in Guerlain's Guet-Apens? This fragrance was designed to claim a great inheritance, and it fits in the family portrait perfectly. Elsewhere, LT compared its beauty to Grace Kelly lighting up the room in

Rear Window. Yet Kelly's beauty lacked content. Compare hers to the melancholy sensuality of Rita Hayworth (or Baghari), the girlish ferocity of Bette Davis (Jolie Madame), or the carnivorous threat of Ava Gardner (Tabac Blond). I find 31 Rue Cambon lovely but not moving because not strange. But perhaps it's just not strong enough. While writing this, I've had to cram my wrist to my nose to smell it at all. Rumor has it that Chanel is hard at work formulating a parfum: let's hope they make it richer and more definite in character. I suspect this slightly inchoate thing could be coaxed into greatness. In the meantime, try on fabric to slow the slideshow. T S

100% Love (S-Perfume) *chocolate rose* $$$
In case anyone still wondered, given the stellar record of great perfume impresarios like Vera Strubi (Angel) and Chantal Roos (Opium), niche firms have demonstrated beyond doubt how important art direction is to getting a perfume right. A well-funded perfume lover may be able to convince talented perfumers to compose for his firm, but mere artistic freedom and a large budget seldom give rise to great perfumes unless the composers are given an idea to work toward and are held to it through what can be a long and painful editing process. Nobi Shioya (his artistic nom de guerre is Sacré Nobi), though we have never met, strikes me from his works as a guy who desires things that are far from obvious and does not rest until he gets them. 100% Love is a case in point. It was lovely in the first version, but clearly not enough. The great, the trismegista Sophia Grojsman recomposed it after only a couple of years. Maybe my day job as a scientist has led me to put too high a value on the novel and the unexpected, but I must say that very seldom (in fact not since 1992) have I had such a

feeling of surprise and delighted incomprehension when first smelling a fragrance. Oddness is easy to achieve—there are many accords nobody ever made—and coziness and comfort too, provided one sticks to the featherbed materials of perfumery: rose, vanilla, chocolate, etc. But to achieve both superlative oddness and mind-numbing comfort at the same time is pure brilliance. If there is a parallel universe in which smells are theorems, 100% Love would be something like a proof of Riemann's conjecture. LT

1740 (Histoires de Parfums) *leather immortelle* $$$
Familiarity with too many trivial perfumes can at length turn one into a libertine of smell: cynical, unmoved, cruelly practical. But every old roué hides at his core an unblemished memory of the boy he once was, ready to fall for the first creature whose intelligence revives his freeze-dried heart. I felt something give way when I smelled 1740: the shimmering classical accord of leather, immortelle, spice, rich pipe tobacco, and a sort of lived-in buttery warmth is simply irresistible. And why resist? LT

2011: Replace pipes and leather slippers with dried roses and raisins and get a sort of Kenzo Jungle thing, not quite the thing we fell in love with. Let's hope the change is a temporary problem of sandalwood supply or similar. TS

L'Air du Désert Marocain (Tauer Perfumes)
incense oriental $$
The sweet smell of amber, the foundation of the classic perfume oriental, has long been weighed down with vanilla and sandalwood, decorated with mulling spices,

bolstered with musk, made come-hither, ready for its close-up, and we are quite used to it—but this is not amber's first life. *Perfume* meant first "through smoke," named for fragrant materials burned to clean the air and therefore the spirit. If, as Carlos Santana claimed in his Grammy acceptance speech, the angel Metatron delivers messages to the world via rock guitarists, it only makes sense that the as-yet-unnamed angel of perfume speaks through an unassuming Swiss chemist from Zurich with a mustache and a buttoned shirt. L'Air du Désert Marocain is talented perfumer Andy Tauer's second fragrance, after the rich oriental rose of Maroc pour Elle. One hale breath of Désert's vast spaces clears the head of all the world's nonsense. There is something about the ancient smell of these resins (styrax, frankincense) that on first inhalation strikes even this suburban American Protestant with no memories of mass as entirely holy, beautiful, purifying, lit without shadow from all sides. Even without the fragrance's name to prompt me, I would still feel the same peace when smelling it that I've felt only once before, when driving across the southwestern desert one morning: all quiet, no human habitation for miles, the upturned bowl of the heavens infinitely high above, and the sage and occasional quail clutching close to the dun earth. Each solitary object stood supersaturated with itself, full to the brim, sure to spill over if subjected to the slightest nudge. Wear this fragrance and feel the cloudless sky rush far away above you. T S

Amouage Gold (Amouage) *huge floral* $$$$
I love the bold, hybrid idea behind Amouage. The firm was started in 1983 by a senior member of the Omani

royal family to restore the trimillennial tradition of perfume in Oman. With the mixture of local pride and interest in faraway lands that befits an ancient seafaring nation, they called it Amouage, from the Arabic *amwaj* (waves), gallicized to make it sound more like *amour*. I have no idea what Oman perfumery is like today, though I've seen documentaries about Muscat guys spraying on clouds of bespoke mixtures in little shops with evident glee. In any event, twenty years ago Amouage hired the great Guy Robert and gave him a brief most perfumers can only dream of: "Put whatever you like in it, no matter how much it costs." Now called Amouage Gold, a little signed card says mine was made by one Naeema, a nice touch. The old bottle was made of crystal containing 24 percent lead: holding it in your hand made you wonder whether gravitation had suddenly quadrupled. The whole thing was put together in a happy, slightly naive, manifestly handcrafted style, which reminds me of the few really valuable things Russia used to produce, like Red October chocolates, confirming my long-held opinion that Moscow is a big Damascus with snow. The fragrance? Guy Robert describes it in the press pack as the crowning glory of his career, and I agree. Robert is perhaps the most symphonic of the old-school French perfumers still working today, and Gold is his Bruckner's Ninth. This perfume is about texture rather than structure, a hundred flying carpets of scent overlapping each other. It's as if Joy had eloped with Scheherazade for a thousand and one nights of illicit fun. After smelling a skimpy modern thing, Guy Robert once despairingly told me, "Un parfum doit avant tout sentir bon." (A perfume must above all smell good.) With Gold, he put the sultanate's money where his mouth was and produced the richest perfume in existence. Small wonder they used to call the region Arabia Felix. LT

2011: Though the silken background is no longer as rich as the sultanate and the top note is evidently thinner, even if Gold were half as luxurious it would be the most decadent fragrance in this style that money could buy. Lovers of the Arpège and Calèche of old, rejoice! TS

Angel (Thierry Mugler) *fruity patchouli* **$**
The first time I smelled Angel, a flamboyant six-foot-three salesman with the shoulders of a linebacker encased in a baby blue zoot suit leaned over the counter and sprayed me. I recoiled. "Is this a joke?" I thought of it, for years, as possibly the worst thing I had ever smelled. I suffered then from the naive belief that women should smell only like flowers or candy; yet Angel, perversely, smells of both, with the same relation to your average sweet floral as the ten-story-high demonic Stay Puft Marshmallow Man from *Ghostbusters* has to your average fireside toasted sweet.

In that sense, Angel certainly is a joke. Countless perfumes have copied parts of it (for a sample, see Euphoria, Flowerbomb, and Prada), but they mistakenly play it straight. Although Angel is sold as a gourmand for girls, spoken of as if it were a fudge-dipped berry in a confectioner's shop, it's all lies. Look for Angel's Adam's apple: a handsome, resinous, woody patchouli straight out of the pipes-and-leather-slippers realm of men's fragrance, in a head-on collision with a bold blackcurrant (Neocaspirene) and a screechy white floral. These two halves, masculine and feminine, share a camphoraceous (mothball) smell, which gives Angel a covering of unsentimental, icy brightness above its overripe (some say "rotting") rumble. The effect kills the possibility of cloying sweetness, despite megadoses of the cotton-candy smell of ethylmaltol, leaving Angel in a high-energy state of contradiction. Many perfumes are beautiful or pleasant, but how many are exciting? Like a woman in a film who seethes, "He's so annoying!" and marries him in the end, I returned to smell Angel so many times I had to buy it.

When this striking idea proved a hit, it gave perfumers hope that, as once was done with Chypre, they could mask this structure a thousand different ways to create new effects. It doesn't really work, though not for lack of trying. The fruity chypres, leather chypres, floral chypres, green chypres, and so on, smell very different. But the Angel format, combining masculine and feminine, in nearly all cases still smells like Angel no matter what you use from columns A and B. Don't fuss with pretenders. Buy the perverse, brilliant original, but wear it only if you know how to tell the joke properly. T S

Après l'Ondée (Guerlain) *heavenly heliotrope* $$$
The advantages of working with a clean sheet of paper are priceless: see the perfection of the first Windsurfer, the first small jet airliner (the SE-210 Caravelle), and in this case (1906) the first serious heliotropin fragrance. The almond-floral note of heliotropin, so reminiscent of the spring-like powdery pallor of mimosa, demands a certain type of wan radiance, which Après l'Ondée embodies perfectly. But as usual with Guerlain, there is a lot more to it than that. The slightly one-dimensional, cheap feel of heliotropin is offset by a melancholy, powdery iris note. If you left things at this point, you'd have

a first-class funeral, complete with four horses and gray ostrich feathers. But Guerlain suffuses the whole thing with optimistic sunlight by using, as in so many of their classic fragrances, a touch of what a chef would call bouquet de Provence: thyme, rosemary, sage. This discreet hint of earthly pleasures is what makes Après l'Ondée smile through its tears. Among pale, romantic fragrances, only Après l'Ondée has the unresolved but effortless feel of the watery piano chords that make Debussy's pieces (*Images* is exactly contemporary) so poignant. One of the twenty greatest perfumes of all time. LT

2011: The joke built into the original was the dressing-up of cheap heliotropin with wildly expensive iris. Now that one is banned and the other is cheaper, the fragrance smells deliciously of iris. Some of the sweet nostalgia of the original is gone, but it is still very good in a suitably anemic way. In fairness, Guerlain could not have done better. LT

Aromatics Elixir (Clinique) *woody floral* $
Smelling Aromatics Elixir on a strip and especially in the air following a string of "modern" fragrances is like watching Lauren Bacall in *The Big Sleep* after twelve episodes of *Cheers*. The thing fills the room with such a confident presence that it is hard to countenance the fact that Bernard Chant was using the same fragrance materials as everyone else. In his hands everything becomes larger and lighter than life. His trademark structure of a bold herbaceous-patchouli-floral accord buttressed by a chiaroscuro of dozens of related balsamic notes produced very sultry, grown-up fragrances

(see Cabochard and Cinnabar). It works even better when done in the bright, fresh, herbaceous, almost medicinal manner of Aromatics Elixir. AE achieves at once salubrious radiance and luxurious dusk, a balancing act to my knowledge only attained since by Patou's Sublime. A masterpiece. LT

Azurée (Estée Lauder) *citrus leather* $
Why is it that, in my years of collecting and talking about fragrances with other people passionate about the stuff, nobody has ever mentioned Azurée? All those connoisseurs love leather, love pre-eighties perfumery, complain that the classics have been debased by lousy substitutions with cheaper stuff. They weep that Cabochard has had its complicated, stormy bits removed; they mourn the streamlining of Jolie Madame; they cry that Caron has tampered with their Tabac Blond; they sigh that an era has passed. Meanwhile, Estée Lauder, faithful keeper of one of the most consistently high-quality lines of fragrances ever created, falls prey to the usual notion that only the new is worth mentioning, and hides the old stuff under the counter like contraband. We hope these fragrances see more of the light of day after this book comes out. Azurée is a grand, confident leather from 1969 by Bernard Chant, creator of Cabochard and Aromatics Elixir, with some of the surprisingly persistent lemony-woody sunshine of Monsieur Balmain and a soft, dusty, almost grimy leather-chypre heart as comfortable as an old work glove, a fragrance now as good as it's ever been and just about as good as it gets. TS

2007 sample.

Azzaro pour Homme (Azzaro) *anisic lavender* $

The monotheists among us believe there is only one proper genre of masculine fragrance, the fougère, and that its apex was reached with the aromatic fougères of the late 1970s. Some, I among them, believe that the finest aromatic ever was Azzaro pour Homme (1978). You can tell it was a perfume aimed at smart guys: the slogan "Un parfum pour les hommes qui aiment les femmes qui aiment les hommes" is not for the slow-witted. I wore it today for the first time in twenty years, and it felt just as it always did: affable, slightly vulgar, completely unpretentious, and overall just delicious. This fragrance is so good and historically so important that I have met to date six perfumers who claim to have composed it (Gérard Anthony is officially credited), which puts it in the same league as Giorgio and a few others for multiple attribution. Azzaro's other fragrances have mostly been disappointments, but all is forgiven. Just keep making this one. LT

Badgley Mischka (Badgley Mischka)
gorgeous fruity $$

The first time I met Badgley Mischka's fragrance was in a lab bottle tester at Bergdorf Goodman, a few months before its release. Sprayed on a blotter, the first thing that happened was a big, breathtakingly gorgeous fruity top note, which I promptly decided to forget about, since what doesn't have a big fruity top note these days? The second time I smelled it, I sprayed it from the real bottle (a set designer's idea of a classy bottle, with a metal nameplate making it look like an executive paperweight) and was immediately floored by a big, breathtakingly gorgeous fruity top note, with both lushness and freshness, reminding me of juicy edibles at the moment of maximum ripeness before everything goes to brandy—peaches, mangoes, lychees, pineapples—but fruity fragrances aren't my style, so I moved on. The third time I smelled Badgley Mischka, I sprayed it from a new tester for the purpose of writing about it, and the first thing I noticed was a really big, breathtakingly gorgeous fruity top note, but as I was feeling rather academic, having just been complaining about the prevalence of fruity fragrances, I focused instead on its similarities to Angel or Gucci's Rush, its lactonic woody drydown that unfortunately thins at the end, talking to LT about a possible link he smelled to Narciso Rodriguez for Her, and so on. The fourth time I sprayed it, it was after I'd written a dry, appreciative review, calm, sensible, and helpful, and it was evening, after dinner, with the lights out; I wanted to smell that big, gorgeous fruity thing again, now that the pressure was over. It rang out, came chorusing up from the skin in great clear peals like church bells on Easter morning, simple and perfect and sure, a message of straightforward good news, and I imagine it's rather like this when the long-suffering hero looks up at the end of a string of confused romantic disasters only to discover that his longtime friend has all this time been the most beautiful girl in the room, and only familiarity prevented him from seeing it. Time to face the facts and hire a caterer—it's love. T S

Bandit (Robert Piguet) *bitter chypre* $$
I'll start with a note of caution: I've owned several bottles of the original Bandit over the years, and this is not it. But read on. Reproducing modern versions of Germaine Cellier's masterpieces is both easy and hard: easy, because her perfumes had such bold, distinctive structures that

even a pixelated version of Bandit, such as the last, dreadfully cheapened and traduced "original" version, was still recognizably the old scoundrel; hard, because Cellier was fond of using bases in her compositions, to the horror of other perfumers. Bases are mini-perfumes, prepackaged compositions that dispense you from reinventing the wheel every time you need a complex but recognizable note in your fragrance: peach, leather, amber, etc. Some, like Ambre 83, Persicol, and Animalis, are so rich and so good that you wonder why nobody just bottled them and sold them. The problem with Cellier's use of bases is that half of them have disappeared, so that even if the whole formula were to fall into your hands and you trekked to the address of the maker of Dianthiline 12 in Grasse, you'd likely find a time-share development instead of a little fragrance factory. Modern reconstructions of Cellier's perfumes are above all a work of translation of the original formula into things you can actually identify and buy today. In my opinion, this can be positive: these perfumes always carried a certain amount of excess baggage to compensate for the starkness of the basic accord. If it can be done elegantly, a cleanup is in itself no bad thing. One just has to get used to the idea that, as with vintage aircraft, what you see is a machine in which perhaps only the serial number plate subsists from the original, and every spar and rivet has been made from scratch. This version of the 1947 original is a bit like a reconstructed Bell X-1 supersonic aircraft: sleek, beautifully done, and a mite too clean, as if ready for a movie shoot. But the magic is all there: bitter, dark yet fresh, beguiling without any softness, and still several unlit streets ahead of every other leather chypre around. LT

2007 sample.

Beyond Paradise (Estée Lauder) *symphonic floral* $

Perfumery becomes art only when it adds something to nature. Applied to florals, however, this banal statement hides a multitude of tricky technical questions. For a start, many flowers, such as gardenia and lily of the valley, yield no oil, and those that do, like rose, produce materials that bear little resemblance to the real thing. Doing a rose, lily-of-the-valley, or gardenia soliflore is therefore artistically as hard as it gets. But realistic florals, though they may be great achievements, should really be judged by a panel of bees rather than by humans. Women have no business smelling like flowers. Abstraction has always been the soul of great perfumery, and abstract florals, where floralcy is not tied to one flower or another, have contributed many of perfumery's greatest masterpieces—such as when a judicious mixture of jasmine and rose, as in the old Vent Vert or in Joy, immediately achieved a glorious choral effect in which individual voices were lost. Doing abstraction with aromachemicals is both trickier and more interesting. Composing a floral one molecule at a time is a formidable combinatorial task, made possible only because over time the problem, like a really hard theorem, has been split into lemmas tackled by different perfumers, and reduced to groups of materials that achieve this or that effect. The enormous artistic edge that chemistry gives perfumers is the ability, familiar to the gods of Olympus and to fairy godmothers when putting together a titanically gifted baby, to compose a personage from disparate inherited virtues: the rosy, grassy freshness of lily of the valley, the rasp of lily proper, the mushroom note of gardenia, the lemon of magnolia, the banana of ylang-ylang, the deep woody velvet of violets, the boozy sweetness of rose, the soapy edge of cyclamen, etc. Marshaling all these molecular genes into producing something viable, even beautiful, is far from easy. It requires an eye and a nose for both the overall effect and individual detail: each molecule must at different times join up with others in different roles to achieve a graceful arc from top note to drydown. Calice Becker's Beyond Paradise, coming as it does after a series of masterly approximations—her Tommy Girl and J'Adore (respectively, high noon and sunset)—hits to perfection the dappled, fresh light of early morning shining on the sort of impossible garden that Swedenborg would have seen in visions and described in detail. Not sure about Beyond, but definitely Paradise. LT

People who become fixated on perfume, enough to start knowingly buying more than they can actually wear, frequently enter the kingdom through a side door: seeking the strange, the hard-to-find, the pearl beyond price, the long-lost something-or-other. Their minds (and mine, once) tend to go blank when presented with an attractive abstract floral meant to appeal to the hoi polloi. Instead, what the collector of arcana tends to like in florals are legibility, meaning smells you could name from the garden, and imbalance, meaning smells that draw attention to themselves for being outsized or wrong, like avant-garde clothes with unlikely diagonal zippers or puffy volumes where you wouldn't expect. Yet, as I got used to sampling the more recherché florals, a couple of facts eventually emerged from the mass of data: first, as LT points out, balanced abstraction, not representation, is the greater and more difficult art in florals, and second, most florals maintain their illusion only for a brief time, and thin out rapidly or fall apart into constituents, like those sculpture installations of seemingly unrelated objects that from a certain angle spell a word or draw a picture. What is so impressive about Beyond Paradise's masterful portrait of a gorgeously fresh, fictional, ideal tropical flower, possessed of most of the floral virtues, is that the image holds steady for hours of drydown. But the seamless end product doesn't tend to invite consideration of the stubborn perfectionism that must have guided its construction: it takes a lot of work to make something this accomplished appear this easy. Lovers of the exotic beach-fantasy florals put out by numberless niche firms should pick up the weird sci-fi rainbow nipple bottle at the Lauder counter someday and give it an honest try. This said, I confess I admire this fragrance mostly without loving it, which probably says more about me than about Beyond Paradise. I once blurted out about a beautiful, buoyant piece of Mozart's that LT was in the middle of thoroughly enjoying, "You know, man, this thing lacks hip action." At the risk of sounding cranky, my favorite old florals like Joy and Fracas seem all by themselves to conjure up a personal presence in the room, almost solid, someone whose sleeve you might touch. In the last analysis, what often leaves me cold with squeaky-clean BP-style modern florals is that they smell perfect and lovely but not alive—I grasp into space but there's no one there. TS

2007 sample.

Beyond Paradise Men (Estée Lauder) *green woody* $
Never has the word *accord* been more appropriate than for BP Men. The discovery of the citrus-herbaceous note of dihydromyrcenol in the early nineties added a pale gray puzzle piece to fit somewhere at the junction of yellow citrus, blue lavender, and green melon. As long as

differential volatilities are properly taken into account, very complex chords incorporating all these colors can now be created. BP Men is a perfect illustration. What is special about BP Men is the way it works more like music than like fragrance. Wear it, and after a few hours you will find your daily life suffused by the same feeling of peace you get when you settle into an armchair after tidying your apartment from end to end. All other masculines (and most feminines) seem loud, coarse, and bare by comparison. Its composer, Calice Becker, has miraculously found a way to bottle a never-ending dawn such as Concorde pilots used to see when flying westward, racing with the sun. LT

2007 sample.

Black (Bulgari) *hot rubber* $$
Some of the best fragrances in history are built on precarious equilibria between two contrasting ingredients: the vanilla-vetiver accord of Habanita, the citrus-amber of Shalimar. This widens their emotional keyboard and, when the job is properly poised, allows them to smell different from moment to moment and from mood to mood, as if they always had something new and apt to say. In other words, they smell interesting, as opposed to merely beautiful. A friend of mine used to say that one particular type of short-grain Carnaroli rice he used for risotto seemed to understand his intentions and to possess native intelligence. I can now extend this insight to perfume: Black is buzzing with brains. It was composed by one of the greatest talents in the business, Annick Ménardo of Firmenich. Binary accords having been exhausted, what she did was increase the number of dimensions by one. Black sets out boldly into space

on three axes: a big, solid, sweet amber note; a muted fifties Je Reviens floral note (benzylsalicylate) as green as a banker's desk lamp; and finally a bitter-powdery, fresh rubber accord such as one encounters in specialist shops or while repairing a bicycle tire puncture. These three tunes hit you in perfect counterpoint when Black is first put on. The remarkable thing about Black's structure is the absence of top notes or drydown. Ménardo has contrived to make the harmony independent of perfume time, but very sensitive to small variations in one's perception. At different times, Black will strike you variously as a battle hymn for Amazons, emerald green plush fit for Napoleon's box at the Opéra, or just plain sweet and smiling. It also has the combination of great bones and good skin characteristic of old-fashioned perfumery, while being entirely novel and modern. Some things strive to be classics; others simply are. Spend an evening with Black and you will know that its place is with Bandit, Tabac Blond, and Cabochard among the great emancipated fragrances of all time. LT

Bois des Iles (Chanel) *sandalwood oriental* $$$
Anyone who has ever worn real Indian sandalwood oil straight knows that it is a perfume in itself: milky, rosy, ambery, woody, green, marvelous. What Ernest Beaux's plush Cuir de Russie did for leather, his cozy Bois des Iles did for sandalwood. Though I've never worn a sable stole, I insist it must feel like wearing Bois des Iles: a dark, close, velvety warmth, sleepy and collapsingly soft. For once the marketing material has it right. Chanel says it smells like gingerbread in the drydown, and so it does, sweet with vanillic balsams and spice. But that description doesn't begin to communicate the depth of the fra-

grance: there are aldehydes sifting a powdery brightness over all, so that the fragrance feels sometimes like the brunette sibling of No. 5. There is the delicious top note of citrus and rose, with the fruity brightness of a cola. It is basically perfect and, though over eighty years old, seems as ageless as everything Chanel did in those inventive years. If you think of all the best Chanel fragrances as varieties of little black dress—sleek, dependable, perfectly proportioned—Bois des Iles is the one in cashmere. I have worn it on and off for years, whenever I felt I needed extra insulation from the cold world. TS

2011: Some of the comforting mulled-wine softness of the original is gone, replaced by a slightly harsher and hollower, more sugary amber. This was never going to be easy given the restricted availability of sandalwood, but Chanel has done wonderful damage-limitation work, especially in the top and middle notes. LT

Bois de Violette (Serge Lutens) *woody oriental* $$$
Shiseido's Serge Lutens had just finished overseeing the creation of Féminité du Bois, which took its sweet woody cue from Caron's Parfum Sacré, itself derived from Chanel's Bois des Iles: resonant, strings-only chords almost devoid of time evolution. The woody-fruity structure of Féminité was first devised by the perfumer Pierre Bourdon, apparently on a visit to Marrakech, and then passed on to perfumer Chris Sheldrake, who developed it with Lutens looking over his shoulder to keep it as dark and transparent as humanly possible. The result was the fragrance that properly put Shiseido on the map. Unusually, Sheldrake and Bourdon generously credit each other with the basic idea. When Lutens decided to open his fragrance shop in the Jardins du Palais Royal in Paris,

like a publisher he needed several titles to kick off his collection. Enter the technique known as overdosage, widely propagated by Bourdon, in which a backstage component in one perfume is moved to the forefront in a new composition, a sort of rotation in perfume space. From Féminité du Bois came four variations, three of which create new effects by bold-typing one of the components of the original: musk (Bois et Musc), fruit (Bois et Fruits), amber (Bois Oriental). The fourth, Bois de Violette, differs because the woody-fruity violet smell of methyl ionone recapitulates and intensifies the rest of the fragrance. Its rotation takes place around the center; the stained-glass mandala is perfected by a violet gem around which everything dances. I remember stepping out of Lutens's purple shop into the perpetually quiet walled gardens, armed with this purple smell with a purple name, thinking I was carrying the most precious object in the world. Curiously, Bourdon went on to do a fifth variation in a different context. He apparently included one of his Féminité sketches as an afterthought into a presentation for Dior, and to his embarrassment they picked it, resulting in Dolce Vita. LT

2011: Especially in the top notes, the idea is more legible and literal, a still life of pencils and pansies instead of a mysterious abstraction. An enormous lilac seems to have originally smoothed over where cedar joined violet. Without that cover, the workings beneath are all visible. Still great: old and new converge to nearly the same thing after an hour or two. TS

Boucheron (Boucheron) *massive floral* $$
Composed by Jean-Pierre Béthouart (he of Fendi Palazzo) in 1988, this is the Athena Nike of all floral ori-

entals. The genre lends itself to sensory overload and thick orchestral scoring: imagine having at your disposal the combined forces of Joy and Shalimar to play with, and you will see how most perfumers end up with monsters intent on world domination. But there is beauty to be found in that direction, the oversized, heavy beauty of Art Deco marvels: Hoover Dam, Milano Centrale railway station, Moscow State University—stylized grandeur that offsets weight of materials by simplicity of line. When it came out, Boucheron felt like a Firmenich mission statement: we are an aromachemicals manufacturer and can outdo nature as and when we wish. Boucheron, at the time, felt almost 100 percent synthetic and, amazingly, none the worse for it. Being near someone who wears it is like having your picture taken next to a marble foot as big as a car. LT

2011: This one was never going to be easy to slip by the new IFRA rules: lots of citrus materials up top, big slug of jasmine and ylang in the middle, and hard-to-get sandalwood at bottom. The new Boucheron has completely lost the stately density of the old one and is a transparent affair, with a very pleasant tagete-orange blossom accord and a refined, creamy drydown. LT

Breath of God (LUSH) *smoked fruit* $
In 2007, LT reviewed two surprising, beautiful fragrances—Inhale and Exhale—that came in a box with the Parfum d'Empire scents but turned out to be from the now defunct firm Be Never Too Busy to Be Beautiful. According to Simon Constantine, the brand's head of fragrance, he thought to combine the smoky vetiver of one and the delicious alien fruity floral of the other and call the result Breath of God. Such an experiment should

be a hot mess. But it's a triumph, a walk through an autumnal landscape in shades of pencil gray instead of painterly gold, with the sweet biological rot of compost below and dry air touched with woodsmoke above. In structure it is reminiscent of the best of Serge Lutens's scents, straddling the dark cedar-violet of the Bois fragrances and epic florals such as Sarrasins and El Attarine, and it has an herbal air of archaic medicine or potions to ward off malice. Surreal combinations—lemon ham, grape leather, bubblegum tobacco, loquat vetiver—rise from its depths each time it comes to attention, hour after hour. Wearing it, I feel a sense of wonder that so late in the perfume game there still can be such profound invention. T S

2011: After a brief discontinuation, Breath of God is now in good company as part of the excellent new LUSH range of fragrances.

Calandre (Paco Rabanne) *aldehydic floral* $$
Some years ago, the French perfumery world, distressed by the resemblance of Molinard's Nirmala to Angel and the impossibility of copyrighting a (usually secret) formula, tried to set up a commission of experts that would decide when a perfume was a copy. The idea foundered on the Rive Gauche problem: RG came a year after Calandre (1969) and smelled sufficiently similar that even a perfumer could briefly mistake their drydowns in isolation. Nevertheless, RG was in many ways an improvement on Calandre, richer, darker, more complex. Inexplicably, while perfumers were unanimously positive about Rive Gauche, opinions on Calandre went from disparaging (a mess) to fulsome (brilliantly sim-

ple). Events have, in my opinion, worked out in Calandre's favor. The Rive Gauche reformulation(s) have slightly obscured the structure that made it memorable, whereas it remains entire in the less ornate Calandre. Buy lots of it before someone messes with it too. LT

2011: Still remarkably true to form, considering the pressure Paco Rabanne must be under to slash and burn the old formula. Long at the number two spot behind Rive Gauche, now edging clearly ahead of its altered rival, and the only one of the two preserving that priceless accord of rose, spice, and cream. LT

Calyx (Prescriptives) *guava rose* $$
Sometimes, while reviewing yet another middling batch of perfumes and looking in vain for their reasons for being, I wonder if the problem is me, if critical thought has obliterated pleasure at last and my days as a hedonist are through. Naturally, the next bottle is always a stunner. Like all Sophia Grojsman's best works, Calyx is built on a bold, simple structure: fruity (with a high-profile role for the deliciously garbagey, overripe smell of guava) plus floral (powdery rosy) plus green (neroli and oakmoss). From top to bottom, Calyx maintains its perfect balance between clean crispness and rich sweetness without ever falling into either camp completely. Grojsman has a knack for getting an idea absolutely perfect: there's nothing you could add or take away here, like a perfectly tuned choir out of which you cannot distinguish any individual voice. Furthermore, I can't remember another green fragrance so friendly. Chanel's Cristalle, for example, and Gucci's Envy never escape a narrow-eyed bitchy effect. For a scent of the eight-

ies—1986, to be exact—Calyx also manages to smell incredibly fresh and modern, perhaps because it helped inspire the next generation of fruity clean florals, although none have really improved on it. It's one of those rare fragrances you could wear your whole life. T S

Ça Sent Beau (Kenzo) *tangerine fougère* $
There are two known roads to creating a striking, top-notch perfume: do either a virtuoso version of a known classic form (the silk satin ballgown) or a brilliant invention (the Diane von Furstenberg wrap dress). Kenzo's appropriately named Ça Sent Beau (That Smells Beautiful) from 1987 navigates the latter route, thanks to perfumer Françoise Caron, whose earlier Ombre Rose for Jean-Charles Brosseau still stands as proof of the possibility of finding a novel structure using a few simple, familiar materials. Ça Sent Beau's achievement is especially striking when you compare it to Gaultier's Classique, built on similar materials (orange citrus notes and powdery, fresh woody musks): the Gaultier is stonking, costumey, heavy, reminiscent of the laundromat, while the Kenzo is trim, chic, and reminds you of nothing on earth. On a woman, it has an air of cheerful efficiency and charm; on a man, it's a good-humored alternative to Caron's Royal Bain de Champagne, a Brut with fruit. Kindly ignore the bottle, which looks like a plug-in nightlight from the Dollar Store. T S

2007 sample.

Chamade (Guerlain) *powdery floral* $$
I lived near the Champs-Elysées, two streets up from the Guerlain store, when Chamade came out in 1969, and I remember it wafting out of door number 68 as

people came in and out. It was, as someone said of the Concorde, a new shape in the air. In those days I didn't buy perfumes, and initially thought Chamade was two distinct fragrances: I would smell the drydown on passersby and find it wonderful, but it took me months to connect it to the nondescript floral green top note. Chamade is perhaps the last fragrance ever to keep its audience waiting so long while props were moved around behind a heavy curtain. The drydown, when it finally arrived, was beautiful, a strange, moist, powdery yellow narcissus accord that had the oily feel of pollen rubbed between finger and thumb. The modern Chamade still smells great but gets to the point much faster and has a slight flatness I have noticed in recent Jicky versions, something milkier and more sedate in the vanillic background. Nevertheless, a masterpiece. LT

2011: Let me preface this by saying that nothing in recent years has come close to the original 1969 vintage. I have no idea what in the composition went south in the eighties, but by 2005 much of the soft, powdery, slightly oily and extraordinarily tenacious pollen-like effect was already gone. The 2011 completes that process: something has caved in in the middle, and two sustaining pillars are now separated by a gap. On one side, an intense, hissy-green galbanum note; on the other, a floral lactonic accord reminiscent of Dioressence. If you blink, step back, and smell it quickly you can fool yourself into seeing the original shape. Smells good on its own terms, though. LT

Chinatown (Bond No. 9) *gourmand chypre* $$$
The endearingly plucky firm of Bond No. 9 has produced its first and so far only masterpiece. Composed

by the young Aurélien Guichard (son of the great Jean of Roure, now Givaudan), it is one of those fragrances that smells so immediately, compellingly, irresistibly great that the only sane response is love at first sniff. Chinatown is at once oddly familiar and very surprising, as if the lyrics in a favorite love song had been rearranged to make a new poem, just as affecting but unplanned by the original author. On the one hand, Chinatown harks back to classic, haughty green chypres like Cabochard, Givenchy III, and the first Scherrer. On the other hand, it has an odd, almost medicinal note reminiscent of the mouthwatering dried-fruit smell of Prunol, a base originally composed by Edmond Roudnitska for the defunct firm of De Laire. The combination strikes a precarious but totally convincing balance between remoteness and affability that suggests a personality at once full of charm and dangerous to know. Some people find it too sweet. To my nose it smells like a corner of a small French grocery in summer, in the exact spot where the smell of floor wax meets that of ripe peaches. A treasure in a beautiful bottle. LT

Cool Water (Davidoff) *aromatic fougère* $
This beautiful 1988 composition made Pierre Bourdon famous and was imitated more times, I'll wager, than any other fragrance in history save Chypre. The problem with successful masculines is that you associate them with the legion of aspirational klutzes who wore them for good luck. Trying to assess CW without conjuring up the image of some open-shirted prat with hair gel is a bit like the Russian cure for hiccups: run around the house three times without thinking of the word *wolf*. This said, unlike Chypre, CW belongs to the category of things done right the first time, like the first

Windsurfer and the Boeing 707. Countless imitations, extensions, variations, and complications failed to improve on it or add a jot of interest to this cheerful, abstract, cheap, and lethally effective formula of crab apple, woody citrus, amber, and musk. Now let women wear it for a decade or two. LT

Cristalle (Chanel) *citrus chypre* $$
Fragrance taxonomist Michael Edwards, whose classification eclipses all others, puts Cristalle among the crisp citruses. This is unquestionably correct, but what makes Cristalle fascinating, like an intermediate life-form that shows evolution midway through morphing from one species to another, is that it also belongs somewhere in the green chypres (fresh mossy wood in Edwards's scheme). Considered as a citrus, Cristalle is far too solemn. Considered as a chypre, it has an unusual morning (possibly morning-after) feeling. There is a business-like briskness that suggests waking up from a night spent with a gorgeous stranger and finding her fully dressed and made up, ready to leave after nothing more than a peck on the cheek, leaving only a cloud of Cristalle as a contact address. Beautiful, and a little scary. LT

2011: The edgy beauty of the galbanum-citrus top note, a sort of icosahedral lemon, is now sharp enough to cut paper, shape unchanged. My discreet inquiries lead me to believe there has been a modification in the quality of the galbanum, for once for the better. Magnificent as ever. LT

Cuir de Russie (Chanel) *leather luxury* $$$
Leather notes in perfumery are due chiefly to two raw materials, smoky rectified birch tar and inky isoquino-

lines, the first natural and the second synthetic. They are not necessarily used together, and Cuir de Russie includes only the former. *Rectified* is a polite word for "cooked," and to this day in places such as Russia and Canada where birch is abundant, the sap is cooked in large pans until it turns black and fragrant. The results are pretty variable, but always deliciously complex: a lot of chemistry happens in a few minutes when things roast. Sadly, the use of birch tar is now restricted by the European Union, and I was afraid of what this would do to Cuir de Russie. The answer is not much. This superb fragrance still smells exactly as it should: to me, just like the interior of my stepfather's 1954 Bentley Type R, in the back of which I sat alone as a child, toying with the mahogany fold-out table on the seat backs. What is remarkable is that this rich leather effect is achieved by mixing things that have nothing to do with tanned animal skins: ylang, jasmine, iris, all of which can be perceived in the top notes. There have been many other fragrances called Cuir de Russie, every one either too sweet or too smoky. This one is the real deal, an undamaged monument of classical perfumery, and the purest emanation of luxury ever captured in a bottle. LT

2011: The smokiness is less sweet and a touch less animalic, as if the birch tar had been partially replaced with something cleaner, more charcoal-like, such as cypriol. There is also a mite less powdery sweetness in the core, probably due to sandalwood adjustments. Overall the fragrance seems a little more spry and masculine. LT

Derby (Guerlain) *smoky wood* $$$
Derby is an oddity, the only case of a Guerlain masterpiece gone unnoticed. Released in 1985, it had very little

impact, probably because of poor advertising and an ugly bottle. It was then repackaged and sold only at the Paris store, then briefly deleted, then reissued and now part of their lineup, one hopes permanently. Guerlain's gush and guff would have us believe that every one of Jean-Paul Guerlain's best fragrances is a paean to the *éternel féminin*. The truth is he's always been rather better at composing things for his own use, exhibits being Vetiver and Habit Rouge. Derby sits halfway between the confident swagger of HR and the dry restraint of Vetiver, on what might be described as the center of gravity of male fragrance. In structure, it is woody-balsamic with a touch of smoke. In radiance, it is like a Kirlian photograph of a healthy leaf, projecting a deep-green aura no farther than an inch, but suprisingly intense and durable up close. One of the ten best masculines of all time. LT

Diorella (Dior) *woody citrus* $$
Diorella came out in 1972, six years after Eau Sauvage, and has all the hallmarks of Roudnitska's mature style, as evidenced in Parfum de Thérèse: a rich, woody-floral accord at once sweet and bracing, very abstract and of no definite sex. I was trying to define the Roudnitska signature for myself, and all I could come up with was that it smelled like herbs, vitamin B, and lime. I didn't dare say it, but it had something oddly meaty about it. I asked my coauthor, "If Guerlain were dessert, which course would Diorella be?" TS was unfazed: "Vietnamese beef salad," she said, which in my opinion is both sacrilegious and exactly right. Diorella was intended as a feminine and was the very essence of bohemian chic, with an odd, overripe melon effect that still feels both elegant and decadent. The modern version, no doubt

fully compliant with all relevant health-and-safety edicts since the fall of the Roman Empire, is drier and more masculine than of old, no bad thing since I have always seen it as a perfected Eau Sauvage and one of the best masculines money can buy. LT

2011: Perhaps all one can do is write futile teary letters asking if it is possible to buy, quietly, gallons of the old forbidden stuff under the table, as if it were scandalous, morally questionable contraband, like dolphin liver pâté. This once exceptional fragrance, both acid-sharp and a little sleazy, was formed of a delicious citrus so rich it was nearly greasy, an unabashedly meretricious jasmine, the austere bitterness of oakmoss, a slice of melon for garnish, and throughout a suspicion of dirty drawers. No one can blame Dior's head perfumer, François Demachy, for allergen regulations that have made citrus, jasmine, and oakmoss tricky to use. While the pleasant greenish lemon tea he has concocted may have some ghost of old Diorella about it, you will need imagination to see it. TS

Dior Homme (Dior) *fruity iris* $$$
The Dior Homme bottle is strikingly solid, more beautifully made than one would expect. In fact, it is good enough to house a feminine perfume. This is quality stuff, and Dior Homme's then man in charge, Hedi Slimane, wanted everyone to know. The fragrance? Composed by Olivier Polge, son of Chanel's Jacques, it takes its place among the half-dozen best masculines of the last ten years. In structure, it flirts with the virtuoso modernist complexity of Hugo Boss's Baldessarini and the muted candied-fruit colors of Chanel's Egoïste. Where it differs is in an interesting, powder-gray iris top

note and a drydown like an attenuated version of Chance with more tobacco. Refined, comfortable, and most of all a textbook example of successful top-down design. LT

2011: Always a marvelous mixture of cheap and expensive, either there is something more flirtatiously creamy and powdery in the woods and musks here, giving this dandified iris more of an old-fashioned barbershop air than before, or I'm just getting sentimental. Great. TS

Dune (Dior) *fresh oriental* $
Forget suburban-gothic names, forget all the phony "noirs," from Angélique to Orris. True, menacing darkness is not to be found in upset-the-parents Alice Cooper poses, but in this disenchanted, ladylike gem. Loosely inspired by the excellent Venise five years earlier (Yves Rocher, 1986), Dune is a strong contender for Bleakest Beauty in all of perfumery. It is clearly headed from the very start toward that peculiarly inedible cheap-chocolate drydown that made Must, Allure (q.v. for a fuller account of the effect), and a thousand others, though Dune's is the best of the lot, dissonant but interesting. But the way it gets there is extraordinary, with a beguiling transparency, even freshness, particularly in the anisic carrot-seed top notes. It is hard to pin down what makes Dune so unsmiling from top to bottom: it's as if every perfumery accord had become a Ligeti cluster chord, drained of life, flesh-toned in the creepy way of artificial limbs, not real ones. Marvelous. LT

2011: The top note is now a plasticky fruity floral. But no worries: after a few minutes, you are back in the familiar, flat, still miles of it, dimmed by unbroken low cloud. TS

Dzing! (L'Artisan Parfumeur) *vanilla cardboard* $$$

Olivia Giacobetti is here at her imaginative, humorous best, and Dzing! is a masterpiece. Dzing! smells of paper, and you can spend a good while trying to figure out whether it is packing cardboard, kraft wrapping paper, envelopes while you lick the glue, old books, or something else. I have no idea whether this was the objective, but I have a few clues as to why it happened. Lignin, the stuff that prevents all trees from adopting the weeping habit, is a polymer made up of units that are closely related to vanillin. When made into paper and stored for years, it breaks down and smells good. Which is how divine providence has arranged for secondhand bookstores to smell like good-quality vanilla absolute, subliminally stoking a hunger for knowledge in all of us. LT

2011: Rumors of Dzing!'s demise were exaggerated. The far drydown has always been a little disappointing, settling on a thin woody thing that says, "Aftershave." But as the top and middle are so delicious, I have always opted to spray it on a scarf or sleeve I can change out of later. TS

Eau de Guerlain (Guerlain) *citrus verbena* $$$$

Eau de Guerlain is to citrus what the mandolin, with its doubled-up strings, is to a guitar. It is as if, by some arcane miracle of perfumery, the ivory and green notes of citron and verbena have been made to sing in harmony with the jaunty lemon-bergamot tune exactly a major third on either side, giving the whole thing a ravishing, nostalgic timbre. Even more miraculous, Eau de Guerlain has a coherent, fresh drydown that completely transcends the cologne genre. If you want citrus, there is simply nothing better out there. LT

2011: EU restrictions on citrus have mandated the removal of photosensitizer furocoumarins, and the cleaned-up oils smell different. The effect of the original accord is still there, but slightly harsher and less well rounded. LT

Eau Sauvage (Dior) *citrus floral* $
I always forget how good this darned thing is. Part of the reason I don't wear it is that it reminds me of my youth. Also, it is a touch louder than I feel comfortable with. Eau Sauvage broadcasts itself quite far by being written in an intrinsically legible type, a sort of Garamond of smell. Great perfumers play with the cologne idea the way Prokofiev used eighteenth-century structures in his First Symphony: take the familiar and, as if it were one of those Transformers my son plays with, turn the horse-drawn carriage into a spaceship. What Roudnitska did to cologne here is threefold: (1) Add a slug of a pine-needles-and-rosemary accord, which the Italians did so well in postwar marvels like Acqua di Selva and Pino Silvestre. (2) Use his own trademark Vietnamese-salad accord (see Diorella for a fuller account). (3) Famously be the first to lubricate the whole thing with hedione, a floral material that can wet the driest lips. I've heard perfumers say there is so little hedione in Eau Sauvage that attributing ES's success to it was a bit like attributing Jascha Heifetz's skill to the Guarneri he played. Either way, a masterpiece. LT

2011: The entire heart has fallen out of this fragrance. It is now close to Jo Malone's Lime Basil & Mandarin, a perfectly nice refined light citrus but no longer in the least bit Sauvage. T S

Enlèvement au Sérail (Parfums MDCI)
peach jasmine $$$$
Despite the silly name (Abduction in the Seraglio, after Mozart's opera), I love this fragrance, and sprayed it several times while writing this review to rewind it to the beginning and see the title sequence again, for it is stunning. It starts with an intensely animalic floral top note; moves on to a golden, seraphic chord of jasmine and peach in the fifties-revival manner of 31 Rue Cambon (which, to be fair, came five years later); and gradually settles to a classical, well-poised voice with a hint of a spicy-woody rasp. You'll probably want to spray it on fabric to admire the graceful trajectory in slow motion. L T

Envy (Gucci) *green floral* $$
Maurice Roucel has a knack for putting together perfumes that feel haunted by the ghostly presence of a woman: Lyra was a compact, husky-voiced Parisienne, Tocade a tanned, free-as-air Amazon. These have another Roucel hallmark, the spontaneity of the unpolished gem. When subjected to the full grind of the marketing department, Roucel's style can become cramped and tends toward brilliant pastiches of classical fragrances: 24, Faubourg; L'Instant; Insolence. Envy is to my knowledge the only time when the balance between Roucel's magic and the real world gave rise to a work that, like a diamond, needed both heat and pressure to form. My recollection is that Envy was panel-tested again and again while Roucel adjusted it until it outperformed Pleasures, then at the top of its arc of fame. It is amusing to think that such a comparison be-

tween apples and pears could be expected to be meaningful. However, it did constrain the woman inside Envy to be at once seraphic and suburban, complete with the sort of suppressed anger that such a creature would feel at being reincarnated as a florist in eastern New Jersey. LT

Le Feu d'Issey (Issey Miyake) *milky rose* $$

The surprise effect of Le Feu d'Issey is total. Smelling it is like pressing the play button on a frantic video clip of unconnected objects that fly past one's nose at warp speed: fresh baguette, lime peel, clean wet linen, shower soap, hot stone, salty skin, even a fleeting touch of vitamin B pills, and no doubt a few other UFOs that this reviewer failed to catch the first few times. Whoever did this has that rarest of qualities in perfumery, a sense of humor. Bravo to those who did not recoil in horror at something so original and agreed to bottle it and sell it, but shame also, since they lost their nerve and discontinued it before it caught on. Whether you wear it or not, if you can find it, it should be in your collection as a reminder that perfume is, among other things, the most portable form of intelligence. LT

Still discontinued.

Fracas (Robert Piguet) *butter tuberose* $$$

A friend once explained to me how Ferrari achieves that gorgeous red: first paint the car silver, then six coats of red, then a coat of transparent pink varnish. Germaine Cellier would have approved. Her masterpiece Fracas, after going through a threadbare patch in the eighties, was revived by a U.S. outfit and spruced up to a quality approximating the original as far as possible, with the usual Cellier caveats of disappeared bases (see Bandit). To my nose, what makes Fracas great is a wonderful buttery note up top, which I attribute to chamomile, and a nice bread-like iris touch in the drydown. Pink and silver, with tuberose red in between. LT

2011. Even better. TS

Givenchy III (Givenchy) *green chypre* $$$
An earthy English friend of mine used to be fond of the expression "good, clean dirt," which she applied to situations that would have sent most people scurrying for tetanus shots. She would have loved this spruced-up reissue of G III: the leather and green chypres all have a curious lived-in quality that gives Bandit, Jolie Madame, and even the rather prim Y a special feel, as if one were simultaneously smelling several successive applications of the same fragrance on fabric without a dry-clean in between. G III was always the brightest and soapiest of the lot, but it still retained a faintly morning-after atmosphere. This long-awaited reissue is a wonderful thing, quite a bit drier and lighter than the original but none the worse for it, and quicker getting into the distinctive strings-only leafy-green heart, which goes on forever. Excellent, and a great masculine too. LT

2011: Now it resembles the far drydown of a nameless vintage fragrance, as if you'd broken open an unmarked plastene sample tube from some forgotten fifties drug-store delight. The oakmoss has been quieted; the floral is gone; there is a pleasant smell of hot radio, a bit of celery seed, and a suave musk, not much else. Still a great masculine but too subdued to compete with the great feminines. TS

Grey Flannel (Geoffrey Beene) *sweet green* $

Very few masculines have been more influential than GF, released in 1975. It is the halfway stop in the long journey that leads from Fougère Royale to Fahrenheit. While still properly herbaceous and inedible, its distinguishing feature is a top note in which fresh citrus components were married to the leafy green of violet leaf and galbanum resin in such a way that the fruit-juice quality of the citrus was completely gone, and only its woody aspect survived. This weird accord was a precursor of the woody almost-citrus (dihydromyrcenol) of Cool Water, only far richer. What makes GF fascinating is the way the dry half of the fragrance is rounded off by a sweet-herbaceous coumarinic note that provides perfect balance and fit. All in all, and despite the fact that GF can occasionally feel a little crude, a masterpiece. LT

Habit Rouge (Guerlain) *sweet dust* $$

One of the most immediately and permanently appealing ideas in all of perfumery, the orange-flower-and-opopanax accord, soft and rasping like stubble on a handsome cheek, is a bit like beauty itself: immediately understood, never quite elucidated. The new version of HR, which may have undergone some cleanup at the hands of Edouard Fléchier, appears sparer, less laden with dandified frippery than previous ones. This emphasizes HR's most attractive aspect, the surprising but in retrospect self-evident character that is the hallmark of a work of genius. LT

2011: This one poses a Heraclitean question: does one ever spray on the same Habit Rouge twice? The 2007 version had already jettisoned some of the *vieux beau* sweetness of the original, which as a young man I was fond of but eventually found tiresome and hard to carry off. The new version goes further still in removing what was left of soft focus, and HR is now a cluster of notes crisply separate but in perfect parade step with each other: dusty leather, dry woods, sweet orange flower, all present and correct. Excellent. LT

L'Heure Bleue (Guerlain) *dessert air* $$
When it comes to arranging a folk theme, the early twentieth century had Mahler and L'Heure Bleue, and we have Enya and Fleurs d'Oranger (L'Artisan Parfumeur, Lutens, etc.). The brilliance of L'Heure Bleue is to cast fresh, shallow, sunny orange flower in a huge role, flanked by two giants: eugenol (cloves, carnation) and ionones (woody violets). Their chorus inexplicably achieves a mouthwatering praliné effect close to that lethal Torino delicacy, the Gianduja. This is Guerlain the virtual pastry chef at his best, with a fragrance that teeters on the edge of the edible for hours without missing a step. If you're Red Hot Riding Hood and a hungry wolf just rang the bell, this is the one for you. LT

2011: A pretty stranger has come in claiming to be your best beloved. It is hard to be angry with her. She is clearly out of her mind; they look nothing alike. You sit and wait patiently for your love to turn up. The windows go dark, night after night while the stranger smiles and dawdles, waiting for you to forget. Can you? TS

Homage (Amouage) *incense rose* $$$$
At the impossibly swank launch in Muscat of Amouage's two Jubilation scents, guests found, upon arrival in their hotel rooms, a limited edition bottle in a plain white box

labeled simply Attar; i.e., "fragrance." When sampled, this anonymous thing turned out to be breathtakingly beautiful: at once lofty, tremendously radiant, and dizzyingly rich. Faced with such an apparition, most of us immediately look around for someone to share our impressions, and the more witnesses the better. I felt the usual mixture of pride and frustration at being in possession of a thing of beauty that few others could share. For company, I gave some to my eight-year-old daughter, who wears it on big occasions. Thankfully, this mysterious Attar, renamed Homage, is now available in limited distribution. The firm tells me it was composed in-house, chiefly of Cambodian oud, Ta'if rose, and Omani silver frankincense, which is to say, the best and most expensive stuff around. Oman was making perfumes when Europeans only bathed once a year on doctor's orders. While there, I had occasion to sample, both in shops and in the wake of passing Omanis, the local style of oud, a fiercely elegant accord of rose and wood that radiates aquiline beauty. For Homage, the firm has gone one better on the usual composition and added not only frankincense, which fills the composition with stratospheric light and ice, but apparently some citrus oils to make it more pleasing to Western noses. Mine finds it irresistible. LT

Insensé (Givenchy) *masculine floral* $$
Insensé is back! Givenchy must be commended for bravely reissuing marvels from its distinguished past, not least because they put most of its present offerings to shame. The reissues of III and Vetyver were a great idea, since the world cannot have too many vetivers and green chypres. But Insensé was a matter of far greater import.

When it was released in 1993, it was one of the most original masculines in decades and that rarest thing, a floral for men. Michael Edwards's database lists only eight such (leaving aside lavenders), a tiny number if you consider that there are 659 aromatic fougères. Insensé was far too clever for its time, and bombed miserably, hindered by a wan, floppy-haired, bloodless advertising image that suggested it was a perfume for wusses. And in retrospect you can see why: despite doomed attempts to swim upriver, such as Globe (Rochas) and No. 3 (Caron), the early nineties were going in a completely different, far easier direction, toward spices and woods. Insensé is a remote relative of green chypres. Its composition is unusually complex and hovers between the herbaceous and the green-floral against a woody background, with a touch of the sweet musky character of Rabanne pour Homme. It is blessed with two qualities that are the surest mark of a good masculine: melancholy and mystery. It will likely flop again, so buy it now before Givenchy changes its mind. LT

2007 sample. Given what has happened to Le 3e Homme, it would be surprising for Insensé to still be the same, but I am open to good news. TS

Insolence eau de parfum (Guerlain)
Godzilla floral $$$
In their haste to copy Angel, most perfume houses lost track of the fact that what made it great was not just the smell—that weird combination of patchouli, candyfloss, and blackcurrant—but the effect, the ta-da! moment, the euphoric surprise that a perfume could be so outrageous and still win. The first Insolence came close, except that the shock was spoiled by a violet-hair-spray

top note that made it stumble as it cartwheeled onto the stage. When Guerlain PR offered to send me the new Insolence EdP, I inquired whether the formula was different. The young lady on the phone said yes with a knowing chuckle. And, by golly, it really is different. Guerlain has finally decided that this thing should not even try to be classy and has embraced it as the most deliciously vulgar perfume on the market today. Maurice Roucel's serious compositions are always complex, but there is so much going on here that it feels like a seventies action-movie poster, with a helicopter hovering over a burning building to the right, two cars jumping off a pier in the middle, a girl in a white dress being lifted out of a swamp in a guy's arms at left, and an erupting volcano in the background. The accord is tuberose, red fruit, orange blossom, and a green-peppery Poême-type note that fits perfectly in this context. All four are heavy hitters, and the combination is simply huge. There is something reckless, irreversible, cataclysmic about pressing the spray button on Insolence EdP, even when it is pointed well away from you. I put some on a smelling strip, left it on the table, and walked out for lunch. The perfume ran after me: enough had strayed onto the back of my hand to create a cloud of pink-neon trashiness that made me feel I was being driven to the local café in a stretch limo. When I came back, the strip greeted me heartily across the room. I know I will regret saying this (especially sitting next to it at dinners and concerts), but this Insolence is a masterpiece. LT

Invasion Barbare (Parfums MDCI) *spicy woody* $$$$
This is the first fragrance by Stéphanie Bakouche, graduate of the French perfume school, ISIPCA, student of Patou's former magus Jean Kerléo, and clearly a talent to

watch. On first impression, IB had one of those majestic woody-spicy baritone top notes that usually make me cringe in anticipation that the impressive breadth will soon run out of cash and give way to a skeletal drydown. After ten minutes I uncurled my toes and relaxed: this thing was not done on the cheap, and is in fact one of the top two or three fragrances in this genre on the face of the earth. The closest thing it brings to mind is Penhaligon's old and discontinued Lords, but IB is much better. If you want a distinctive, high-quality masculine less dandified than Mouchoir de Monsieur and less affable than New York, this is it. LT

Iris Silver Mist (Serge Lutens) *iris root* $$$
Long before everybody started doing irises and (mostly) pseudo-irises, Lutens had commissioned an iris to end them all from Maurice Roucel. The story goes that Lutens pestered the perfumer to turn up the iris volume to the max, and Roucel in desperation decided to put in the formula every material on his database that had the iris descriptor attached to it, including a seldom-used, brutal iris nitrile called Irival. The result was the powderiest, rootiest, most sinister iris imaginable, a huge gray ostrich-feather boa to wear with purple dévoré velvet at a poet's funeral. LT

2011: Less brutal, arguably more natural but oddly thinner, more bread-like (iris smells like yeast fumes at times). Something has been lost in translation. A slightly sour floral base creeps up in the drydown. A good iris, but no longer the *monstre sacré* of yore. LT

Jicky (Guerlain) *lavender vanilla* $
Jicky is the oldest perfume in continuous existence: since 1889, the year of the Eiffel Tower, the Exposition

Universelle, the first centenary of the French Revolution. This claim is occasionally disputed by phony pretenders to the throne, like Penhaligon's, Floris, and Houbigant (old names, new formulas) or complete fabrications like Rancé. Such durability cannot be a mere matter of luck: Jicky brought something new to perfumery, and that something still matters today, partly because much that has happened in between is far from good news. By the standards of postwar fragrance, Jicky is a marvel of simplicity, an object lesson in perfumery. The basic idea is lavender and vanilla. Lavender, then as now, was steam-distilled and not wildly expensive. Vanilla is another matter. When Jicky was being conceived, synthetic vanillin made by the Reimer-Tiemann process was just coming onstream, and the firm of De Laire in France had got the license on the patent. The first synthetic vanillin wasn't just cheap; it was different from the natural stuff, far sweeter and creamier. Aimé Guerlain wisely chose a mixture of synthetic and natural, one for power, the other for bloom. But De Laire's yellow vanillin was peculiar, because the German process left a small amount of cough-mixture guaiacol and other smoky phenols in the final mix, which is why Guerlain continued to ask for this special impure grade when the process was improved. Nowadays they just add a touch of rectified birch tar to get the effect. That effect is what Ernest Beaux hankered after when he complained that his vanillas always turned out like crème anglaise, and Guerlain's like Jicky. But vanilla and lavender are only part of the story. Jicky also contains a huge citrus note (think lemon cheesecake), Guerlain's trademark bouquet of French herbs (thyme, etc.), a big dose of civet and Lord (actually Jean-Paul Guerlain) only knows what else. Is the modern Jicky identical to the first one? Of course not. Is it an honest attempt to continue it? Yes. I cannot comment on pre-WWII Jicky, having smelled it only once, and then fleetingly. I can vouch for the fact that the Jicky of my childhood was raunchier, more curvaceous, less stately. What happened? Hard to say: it can't be the lavender or the vanilla, it can't be the citrus, the herbs, or the civet. As Holmes said, "When you have eliminated the impossible, whatever remains, however improbable, must be the truth." My guess is that what made the old Jicky smile were the irreplaceable nitro musks, most of which disappeared from European perfumery years ago because of alleged neurotoxic and photochemical problems. The modern Jicky is perhaps a touch smoother and cleaner than it really should be, but still a towering masterpiece. And one more thing: lest anyone think that unisex perfumes are a modern invention, this one was worn by both women and men ten years before an electric car, the Jamais Contente, broke the world speed record and hit 100 km per hour. LT

2011: Seems punchier, more animalic, richer than the 2007 version. LT

Joy parfum (Jean Patou) *symphonic floral* $$$
There has been much talk about Joy being damaged by reformulation, and I have more than once been called names by Joy aficionados who swear blind that Joy has been changed and therefore I must be either corrupt or incompetent. Nothing is certain in this valley of tears, and Joy may one day be changed, so stock up as if your life depends on it. But the sample of Joy I received in

October 2007 straight from the Patou fountain smelled every last bit as good as it ever did, i.e., sensational. To call Joy a floral is to misunderstand it, since the whole point of its formula (Henri Alméras, 1930) was to achieve the platonic idea of a flower, not one particular earthly manifestation. Joy does not smell of rose, jasmine, ylang, or tuberose. It just smells huge, luscious, and utterly wonderful. LT

2011: In light of European allergen restrictions on jasmine, Jean-Michel Duriez, head perfumer at Patou, must have lost a lot of sleep asking what would become of Joy, the greatest jasmine-rose duet of all time. His answer is in: a perfect rose. The indolic jasmine has mostly gone and taken some lovely civet filth with her. The rose left is even soapier, fruitier, lemonier, greener than before, everything a classic rose wants to be, times ten, all by itself for astonishing hours. As Luca said when I put it on, "It's not Joy, but it's not sadness, either." The new eau de parfum, always a slightly different composition, may even resemble the original more than the current parfum does since in dilution it's easier to meet jasmine restrictions in the final product. TS

Knize Ten (Knize) *amber leather* $$

As Alphonse Allais put it, "As time passes, one meets fewer and fewer people who knew Napoléon." Knize Ten, like the sole veteran of the Grande Armée who lived long enough to be photographed, must feel terribly lonely these days, for it is the only survivor of the androgynous, reckless, dandified twenties leathers. Its elder by five years, Tabac Blond (1919), recently died a death at the hands of International Fragrance Association regulations and Caron perfumer Richard Fraysse, and if you look around there are no pre-WWII leathers left standing: Kobako, Shocking, and no doubt many others, all gone. (Cuir de Russie does not count in this context, because it is primarily a stupendous iris floral with a leather accent.) Knize Ten was composed by François Coty and Vincent Roubert, respectively the man who invented all perfumery and the man who did Iris Gris. For a long period KT was out of stock, and the firm did not know when it would come back, etc. I feared the worst. I cannot vouch for the exact resemblance of today's formula to the original. What I can say is (a) it smells wonderful, with all the proper requisites of a leather, including smoky and amber notes firmly in place; (b) it contains a splendid strawberry top note, which, by a classic piece of perfumery misdirection, kisses you on the lips just as you focus on the dry, dark background; (c) it goes on forever in a completely civilized manner; and (d) it does not cost the earth. Let me put it simply: everyone should own this perfume, because there is only one like it. LT

2011: More floral and even better. This great leather and Cuir de Russie always erred toward the softer and sweeter, to their advantage. TS

Knowing (Estée Lauder) *mossy rose* $
Of all the big fruity roses from the seventies and eighties, Knowing is perhaps the most polished and most wearable. At the time, synthetic fruity rose materials like damascones and damascenones had changed the landscape of rose perfumes, making them bigger, brighter, stronger, practically glow-in-the-dark. The great idea of the rose chypres, beginning with the now-

discontinued Sinan, was to set these intense materials against a classic resinous mossy base—rubies against green velvet—to make these mutant roses seem more civilized and less like the rose that ate Tokyo. The results were striking but sometimes exhausting in their power. Knowing (1988) came late in the game and learned the lessons of its ancestors: it piles on the mossy, woody stuff and lets the pink simply peek out. Worn in small doses, it's just right. TS

2007 sample.

Kouros (Yves Saint Laurent) *musky fougère* $
Twenty-seven years after its release, the structure of Kouros is still so novel, so immediately recognizable, and so impossible to imitate that it is probably a sporadic case in perfumery. It smells like the tanned skin of a guy with gomina in his hair stepping out of the shower wearing a pre-WWI British dandified fragrance: citrus, flowers, musk. It has that faintly repellent clean-dirty feel of other people's bathrooms, and manages to smell at once scrubbed and promissory of an unmade bed. The fact that all these images are conjured up by a fragrance in itself so consummately abstract is a testimony to the brilliance of its creator, Pierre Bourdon. Such things happen not by accident but only as the work of genius. LT

Lavender (Caldey Island) *perfect lavender* $
Lavender is summer wind made smell, and the best lavender compositions are, in my opinion, the ones from which other elements are absent, and only endlessly blue daylight air remains. Everyone should own one to feel good as needed and as a reminder that, in the numi-

nous words of my perfumer-chemist colleague Roger Duprey, "There is no such thing as an uninteresting ten-carbon alcohol." Lavender consists mostly of one such, linalool, and needs careful handling both during distillation and composition to remain true to its benign nature. Caldey Island Lavender was composed for the business-minded monks of Caldey, South Wales, by Flemish freelance perfumer Hugo Collumbien (now age ninety), and is simply the best lavender soliflore on earth. To find it, Google the name. LT

Lolita Lempicka (Lolita Lempicka) *herbal Angel* $$
With most of the many fragrances based on Thierry Mugler's Angel, the first thing you think on smelling them is "Hello, Angel." Not this time. Perfumer Annick Ménardo found the sole variation that stands on its own. In Angel, a loud fruity-floral accord of jasmine, mango, and blackcurrant, like cleavage set to trumpets, is backed up by a somewhat louche and curiously masculine sweet woody section centered on patchouli. Together they sing a husky-voiced come-on. Lolita Lempicka, the first and best of the post-Angel crowd, keeps the sweet woody stuff but skips the pushup bra; instead, it plays out a fresh anisic melody that begins in salty licorice and modulates through several leafy changes as refreshing as lime soda pop, playing Doris Day to Angel's Peggy Lee. The fragrance is snappy and smart, an ideal accompaniment for flirtatious banter delivered by prim girls in glasses. Furthermore, like Ménardo's Black for Bulgari, Lolita Lempicka is a clever feminine that clever men can easily wear. I once got on a subway train just as a pretty young man stepped off in a cloud of it. If it was his girl-

friend's, I hope he was clever enough to nick it. Bonus: darling bottle. T S

2007 sample.

Loulou (Cacharel) *jasmine oriental* $$

Classified by Michael Edwards as Soft Oriental, var. Rich, which is to say Large Baklava, var. Syrupy, this is a perfume that might be reckoned a little over the top even by a Bombay attarwallah. But the secret of Loulou, worked out by the great master Jean Guichard (how does it feel to be the guy who did Eden, La Nuit, and Asja?), is to add a mysteriously raspy note to the whole composition that makes you want to smell more, not push the plate away. When I first encountered it twenty years ago, it made me think of those Christmas tree balls made of purple glass sprayed with black dust, which look like silk and feel like sandpaper. Do not be misled by the fact that Loulou, when found, is likely to be cheap. This is one of the greats. L T

Missoni (Missoni) *kaleidoscopic floral* $$$

Maurice Roucel has, over the years, proved himself a master of compositions at both ends of the perfume time scale, i.e., harmony and melody. Tocade, his definitive essay in short-form perfumery, rang a single chord with very little time evolution, and was all the more remarkable for achieving a totally novel effect using only well-rehearsed raw materials. His various long-form compositions (24, Faubourg; L'Instant; Insolence) demonstrated a growing mastery of counterpoint, whereby the mind's nose, throughout the fragrance's exposition, could focus on layers floating at different depths. In a conversation some time back Roucel recommended I smell his Missoni, about which he was uncharacteristically positive. When the package came, I marveled at the poverty-stricken ugliness of the bottle, and wondered whether Roucel had once again, as with Alain Delon's Lyra, entrusted his best work to a goofy outfit. It seems Missoni got lucky. I have no idea whether they will still be around in ten years, but I'll make sure I have enough of this perfume to last me a lifetime. This is one of the most accomplished fragrances in years, combining in a uniquely convincing way both the horizontal and vertical elements of a perfume score. At first, you mistake it for an entirely delightful hybrid of Tocade and Beyond Paradise. Seconds later, you realize that it has progressed to another chord, still complete with top notes, heart, and drydown, then to another and another, all spanning a wide but entirely comfortable fresh-to-sweet range, all different. Halfway through, when you least expect it, Missoni springs a stunning modulation to a luminous, almost minty accord. The effect is an uncanny feeling that the perfume is alive, somehow composing itself as it goes along. Most other perfumes are rapidly fading photographs: this one is a movie. LT

Mitsouko (Guerlain) *reference chypre* $$
On every occasion when I am asked to name my favorite fragrance, or the best fragrance ever, or the fragrance I would take with me if I had to move to Mars for tax reasons, I always answer Mitsouko. This elicits, broadly speaking, three types of responses: perfumers yawn, beginners write the name down, and aficionados decide I am a staid sort of chap. In truth, it is a bit like saying that your favorite painting is the *Mona Lisa* (not mine, by the way). Mitsouko's history illustrates to perfection the twin forces of innovation and imita-

tion that move perfumery forward. It was released in 1919, supposedly the result of a love affair Jacques Guerlain had with Japan or a lady therein. But there is nothing Japanese about Mitsouko aside from the name. It is, as has been said countless times before, an improvement on François Coty's Chypre, released to huge acclaim two years earlier. Chypre in turn was based on a three-component accord so perfect that it remains unsurpassed and fertile in new developments ninety years later: bergamot, labdanum, and oakmoss. They smell respectively citrus-resinous, sweet-amber-resinous, and bitter-resinous. Picture them as equal sectors making up a pie chart, sticking to each other via the resin. The resulting genre, now called a chypre, has two fundamental qualities: balance and abstraction. Chypre is long gone, but I've had occasion to smell both vintage samples and the Osmothèque reconstruction in Versailles. It is brilliant, but it does have a big-boned, bad-tempered Joan Crawford feel to it, and was a fragrance in whose company you could never entirely rest your weight. Jacques Guerlain was Juan Gris to Coty's Picasso, obsessed with fullness, finish, detail. To Chypre he famously added the peach note of undecalactone, quite a lot of iris, and probably twenty other things we'll never know about. The lactone makes a huge difference: it works like a Tiffany lamp, adds a touch of muted warmth and color, and unlike ester-based fruit notes, lasts forever. The effect of Guerlain's additions is a ripening of the chypre structure into a masterpiece whose richness brings to my mind the mature chamber music of Johannes Brahms. Mitsouko is also a survivor, most recently having dodged a bullet aimed straight at its heart by the European Union's chemical phobia. It looked for a while as if it was going to be reformulated in a hurry. In the end, the great Edouard Fléchier brought Mitsouko into conformity with European Union rules and it still smells great, though it arguably lasts less long than the old one. LT

2011: A faded Art Nouveau poster of the original, with a drydown of one act instead of two, but against big odds, still lovely, still recognizable, and incredibly affecting for it. TS

La Myrrhe (Serge Lutens) *resinous aldehydic* $$$
Judging by the name and the Lutens line, you would think La Myrrhe would be an updated straightforward incense or an amber oriental. Open the bottle and fall prey to total surprise. Gone is the familiar oriental apparatus of spices, vanilla, heavy tobacco, leather, and sandalwood, the whole Cleopatra kit and caboodle. Instead, Lutens and Christopher Sheldrake set the smoky balsamic resin known as myrrh against a radiant, rosy, modern aldehydic floral of incomparable crispness, kin to White Linen. By this unexpected route, the fragrance somehow manages to replicate the thrilling balance of incredible brightness and sweetness that Shalimar once had, before decades of adjustments deepened its voice. La Myrrhe has a pure, clear, unearthly tone with beauty and force, as if the fragrance could sing a clean high C as high as heaven and not show the strain. TS

Nahéma (Guerlain) *virtual rose* $$
The first three minutes of Nahéma are like an explosion played in reverse: a hundred disparate, torn shreds of fragrance propelled by a fierce, accelerating vortex to

coalesce into a perfect form that you fancy would then walk toward you, smiling as if nothing had happened. The consensus among experts is that this fragrance, Guerlain's greatest rose, is in fact done without using any rose at all. Guerlain formulas are usually too rich even for analytical chemistry to make sense of, but from what information can be gleaned, it would seem that the rose at Nahéma's core is a geometric locus bounded by a dozen facets, each due to a different ingredient. Whether that is true or false, accident or skill, it is certainly true that the unearthly radiance of Nahéma is without equal among perfumery roses, and so awe-inspiring that nobody even tries. LT

2011: The latest version reveals how near the edge of the abyss Jean-Paul Guerlain was playing in the original. There has clearly been a small change in the formulation up top, and the vivid original is now borderline garish. Like the camouflage on World War I warships, however, it is still perfectly fine at a distance and with the passage of time. LT

New York (Parfums de Nicolaï) *orange amber* $
If Guerlain had any sense, they would buy Parfums de Nicolaï, add PdN's range to theirs, trash fifteen or so of their own laggard fragrances, a couple of de Nicolaï's, and install owner-creator Patricia de Nicolaï in Orphin as in-house perfumer. She is, after all, a granddaughter of Pierre Guerlain and genetic analysis might usefully reveal the genes associated with her perfumery talent. As a control where the genes are known to be absent, use the DNA of whoever did Creed's Love in White. Smelling New York as I write this, eighteen years after

its release, is like meeting an old high school teacher who had a decisive influence on my life: I may have moved on, but everything it taught me is still there, still precious, and wonderful to revisit. New York's exquisite balance between resinous orange, powdery vanilla, and salubrious woods shimmers from moment to moment, always comfortable but never slack, always present but never loud. It is one of the greatest masculines ever, and probably the one I would save if the house burned down. Reader, I wore it for a decade. LT

2011: Keeping New York identical in the face of both citrus and oakmoss restrictions is beyond the reach of even the most talented, high-minded, and diligent perfumer. Patricia de Nicolaï is all these things, but the new New York is damaged goods. There should be a waiver customers can sign to get the old stuff. LT

No. 5 eau de toilette (Chanel) *peachy floral* $$$
I confess I had until recently failed to understand the differences between the various versions of No. 5. Chanel's engine room tells me that the fragrance has been recast several times over the years, the parfum being the original 1921 formula. This smells like fifties work, with woody-violet notes up top and a lactonic peach drydown. This version is the one I associated with No. 5 all along, largely because I could never afford the others. It is exquisitely beautiful, the true precursor to their recent 31 Rue Cambon, and feels slightly more ladylike than the imperishably crisp real thing. LT

2011: Citrus different, sandalwood different, less smooth and caressing, but still good. Clearly a labor of love in the face of difficult regulatory challenges. LT

No. 5 parfum (Chanel) *powdery floral* $$

When I lived in Villefranche, a little harbor village near Nice, I would occasionally walk to the nearby marina to look at a thirty-foot wooden sloop parked halfway down the pier. It spent most of its life under wraps, surrounded by white fenders. It was one of a pair by a local boatbuilder called Silvestro, his last boat, and had taken fourteen thousand man-hours. When the owner was aboard, you could see it entire. It was more beautiful than an object has any right to be. In fact, it hurt to look at. Other such artifacts: a ladies' black and gray loafer I once saw in Lobb's window in London; the two-thirds-size platinum watch my doctor wears and about which he will reveal nothing; and now, more affordably, Chanel No. 5 parfum. Fragrances very occasionally achieve a compelling 3-D effect, as if you could run your hand along them in midair. The original Rive Gauche and Beyond Paradise are relatively recent examples, but they are still recognizably florals, made of soft, perishable matter. No. 5 is a Brancusi. Alone among fragrances known to me, it gives the irresistible impression of a smooth, continuously curved, gold-colored volume that stretches deliciously, like a sleepy panther, from top note to drydown. Yes, it contains rose, jasmine, and aldehydes in the same way that a perfect body contains legs and arms. But I defy all who smell this to keep enough wits about them to worry about the parts. LT

The beauty and fragrance industry has lied to women for so long, convincing us to fork over cash for crud in shiny packages, that at this point even pure quality has trouble getting taken seriously. Evidence: the persistent and silly question "Has Chanel No. 5 been a best seller because of the fragrance or because of its marketing?" Clever marketing can get us to buy something once, but rarely again. We don't wear Chanel No. 5 because Marilyn Monroe wore it; we wear it for the same reason that Marilyn did: because it's gorgeous. What marked No. 5 as different from its lesser known and largely defunct cousins was an advantageous mutation: an overdose of the bright aromamaterials known as aliphatic aldehydes, harsh alone, but lending an intense, memorable, clean white glow to the rest of the woody floral, which was similar in structure to dozens of others at the time.

Whether, as the legend goes, the slug of aldehydes was a serendipitous mistake on the part of a lab technician preparing a trial, or whether Chanel's perfumer, the brilliant Ernest Beaux, came upon the trick himself, it's impossible to know, but they changed fragrance forever. Yet many more aldehydic florals have entered the market since; they have trickled down to soap formulas to the point that we think of them as the smell of soap. Chanel No. 5 stands out more than ever. Why? Because the firm has done everything in its power to maintain its beauty, even as other famous perfumes have suffered slow attenuation of their former greatness. In a sense, what it once had in common with other fragrances is what helps set it apart now.

Chanel made the wise decision years ago to buy its own jasmine and rose fields and is otherwise known to be fanatic about sourcing materials. Amazingly, despite the fluctuating qualities of natural ingredients from year to year, by careful and constant tweaking, No. 5 continues to smell like No. 5. On my right wrist, I have a No. 5 parfum that predates the fifties, and on my left, a brand-new batch. The musks have changed (wow, those obsolete nitro musks smell grand), and the top notes on the vintage stuff are damaged (smoky off notes, a whiff of burnt butter), but after fifteen minutes these two are nearly the same scent: a masterpiece of modernist sculpture from 1921, one you can wear. It has none of the tasseled-velvet-pillow plush of Shalimar or Vol de Nuit, none of the edgy weirdness of Tabac Blond or Narcisse Noir, none of the drama of Fracas or Bandit. It is an ideally proportioned wonder, all of a piece, smooth to the touch and solid as marble, with no sharp edges and no extraneous fur trimming, a monument of perfect structure and texture. And some people think perfume is not an art. TS

2011: Let it be said that the Chanel crew must have worked shifts to keep No. 5 constant in the face of restrictions or supply difficulties affecting just about everything that goes in it: jasmine, rose, sandalwood, citrus. The fact that the 2011 is even close to what it was is a testament to their skill. Only a weird ketonic note up top, less rich nuttiness in the heart, and less length in the drydown serve to remind us that IFRA are a bunch of traitors. LT

Odalisque (Parfums de Nicolaï) *fresh chypre* $$$
Every once in a long while a composition, steered away from known landmasses by the perfumer's fancy, lands on virgin territory and claims it for itself. What happens afterward depends on the twists of fate, fashion, and finance. Some islands, like Angel, soon attract crowds. Others, like Odalisque, are the Kerguelen Isles of perfumery, unspoiled, windswept, and largely forgotten. Until Patricia de Nicolaï's unerring naviga-

tional sense found it, few would have suspected that land could emerge in the sea between the shy, melancholy, bloodless florals typified by Après l'Ondée and the arch, angular green chypres in the Cristalle manner. And yet there was: Odalisque's superbly judged floral accord of jasmine and iris, both abstract and very stable, allied to a saline note of oakmoss, initially feels delicate, but in use is both sturdy and radiant. It is as if the perfumer had skillfully shaved off material from a classic chypre accord until a marmoreal light shone through it. A unique, underrated marvel, and great on a man as well. LT

Opium (Yves Saint Laurent) *spice king* $
Opium illustrates better than any other fragrance the peculiar phenomenon of love followed by rejection, known as fashion. It is unquestionably one of the greatest fragrances of all time, not only in terms of phenomenal success, but in having deserved it. Yet I would hate it if anyone wore it near me today. Why? Suppose you wrote down the basic requirements for a great fragrance: top of the list would come distinctiveness, then radiance, then (to keep out Amarige-like mutants) some sort of working relationship with natural smells. Opium has the first two in spades and passes muster on the third. But so do Shalimar, Chanel No. 5, and a host of other greats. What is it that makes Opium so dated, when fragrances fifty years older are fresh as paint? I believe the answer hinges on the faults of its qualities. The comparison with its almost exact contemporary and involuntary twin Cinnabar is instructive: both were inspired by the same vision, right down to country (China) and color (vermilion, aka cinnabar). There is something

peculiar about spicy orientals: being made almost entirely of drydown materials, they lack time evolution, the arc of a fragrance that gives it life, and feel like broken wristwatches perennially stuck around 10 p.m. There the resemblance ends. Cinnabar was rich, warm, and fuzzy. Opium said one thing and one thing only, with tremendous force. While this was the most cogent statement ever made by balsams, one does tire of it. This, and not the quality of its raw materials, is what made Opium smell so fascinatingly solid in 1980 and now makes it smell tiresome. LT

2011: Weaker, thinner, and flatter. LT

Or Black (Pascal Morabito) *dark fougère* $$
The firm of Pascal Morabito should not be confused with his parents' outfit, Morabito tout court, which also makes some fragrances. PM makes beautiful steamer trunks in black buffalo leather lined with salmon-colored silk, and the weirdest rings made of something that looks like plastic and is in fact synthetic sapphire encasing a precious stone. He's had these two fragrances (OB and Or Noir) for decades and to my knowledge has done absolutely nothing to promote them, beyond leaving them lying around in his hard-to-find shops. Or Black is an extreme fougère, smoky, dark, bitter, resinous-green, like triple-distilled Earl Grey, a step beyond even Rive Gauche pour Homme in its saturnine glory. Sensational. LT

2007 sample. Michael Edwards, who runs the fragrance database of all databases, lists it as discontinued, but at writing, Pascal Morabito still offers it on their Web site. TS

Ormonde Man (Ormonde Jayne) *green woody* $$

Masculine fragrances (masculine almost everything, come to think of it) rarely venture outside tried and tested stereotypes. Those who try endure the wrath of God. People still shake their heads in disbelief at the brilliantly original Insensé (Givenchy, 1993), "A floral for men . . ." It takes guts to cut loose. Ormonde Man, derived from their signature feminine, is a sultry woody floral that sounds a muted, tourmaline-green chord from top note to drydown. Hear it once, and you'll want it again. L T

Ormonde Woman (Ormonde Jayne) *forest chypre* $$

Of the many feminine perfumes since Bois des Iles that have been composed around woody notes, the others that I can recall have been cozy, powdery-rosy, touched with mulling spices, with the warm furred feeling of a napping cat by the fire, or, more recently, hippie-inspired simple concoctions meant to evoke mostly the gorgeous smell of hard-to-get sandalwood oil. Ormonde Woman is the only abstract woody perfume I know that triggers the basic involuntary reflex, on stepping into a forest, to fill one's lungs to bursting with the air. This is a full-fledged perfume with all the sophistication of Bois des Iles and its ilk, but none of the sleepy comfort. Instead, it has the haunting, outdoors witchiness of tall pines leaning into the night—a bitter oakmoss inkiness, a dry cedar crackle, and a low, delicious, pleading sweet amber, like the call of a faraway candy house. Lulling and unsettling in equal measure, and truly great. T S

Osmanthe Yunnan (Hermès) *milky tea* $$$

When Jean-Claude Elléna, now in-house perfumer at a little saddler's outfit called Hermès, first did the soapy suede-and-apricots scent of the osmanthus flower for The Different Company's Osmanthus, it was like one of those deceptively simple, pretty Paul McCartney melodies that seem so obvious once heard, you suspect he finds them lying fully formed in the street. Elléna could have stopped there. We would have been happy. But instead, in Osmanthus take two, he adds a layer of smoked tea, which could have turned into simply a representation of traditional Chinese osmanthus-scented tea, in itself not a bad idea. But Osmanthe Yunnan also turns up an unexpected milky sweetness at the skin, which transforms what was cool and seen at a distance into something warm and welcoming up close. Put it this way: you'd enjoy Osmanthus wafting by, but you'll follow Osmanthe Yunnan to its source. It is a perfume of pure happiness. If you had asked me before smelling this fragrance if any of the minimalist compositions that Elléna has been turning out in recent years could be ranked in the top tier artistically, I would have said no, by design they'd top out at four stars when at their best; but I would have been wrong. Osmanthe Yunnan is beautiful from start to finish, distinctive, impossible to improve, unforgettable, unpretentious, and the best of Elléna's work for Hermès so far. T S

Oud Cuir d'Arabie (Montale) *leather oud* $$$
Together at last! Oud and leather, two epic, battle-scarred, weather-beaten action heroes of perfumery appear on the same bill. I imagine them pictured against the sun, in ankle-length dust coats, holding a shotgun and a whip, respectively. Full marks to Montale for doing a bite-the-bullet "you sure you want this?" fragrance that sums up all perfumery can offer that's at once rugged, inedible, and lustral. L T

2011: Infected trees give us a vegetal substance, oud, which smells uncannily animal. But as the hours pass, the drydown becomes a spiritual allegory: the beastly bit burns off, the hide falls away, and then emerges a sweet resinous air, not so much strong as fervent. On a man, it is the Clint Eastwood character described by Luca. On a woman, it has unexpected affinities with orientals in the big eighties style of Opium and Red Door, and is at its best the day after, for a leisurely unwashed morning walk home with mascara smeared to your temples like a pharaoh. T S

Patchouli 24 (Le Labo) *strange leather* $$
When I worked summers in the biology department at Moscow State University, there was, at the top of the building, right under the hot roof, a small, airless storage room. Left alone for so long with no company, the vanillic sweetness of the decaying old books had struck up a phenolic conversation with the harsh chemicals in the jars and the fragrant refringent oils in which pickled specimens swam blindly. The smell was at once beguiling, salubrious, and toxic, and felt like a perfume composed for a fiercely intelligent librarian. Annick Ménardo's poetic genius has accidentally re-created that hot, secret space for me. I shall henceforth refer to this fragrance as Labo de Russie. L T

Pleasures (Estée Lauder) *snowy floral* $
In retrospect Pleasures (1995) turns out to have been a tipping point in the history of perfumery, the storming of the fine-fragrance Bastille, the moment when lowly soap finally overthrew the ancien régime and took possession of its empty palaces. Its revolutionary precursors Chanel No. 22 and White Linen illustrate the struggles

of this wish on its way to fulfillment. Aldehydes have always been powerful and cheap, floral bases as well, so soap perfumery made abundant use of low-cost versions of Joy, No. 5, etc. Quality soaps got very good at this, and the advertising (Lux, Camay) started showing demurely bathing blondes up to their necks in white foam worthy of smothering a refinery fire. The soap makers never had the guts to do a fine fragrance scented just like the bar (my prediction is that a Dove EdP would sell well), so it was left to the fine-fragrance people to fake plebeian pleasures. But proper perfume's courtly manners gave it away, and the rose was always too good (White Linen), the musks too sweet (No. 22). By the early nineties two things had happened. First, the relentless impoverishment of fine-fragrance formulas narrowed the gap dangerously with functional fragrance, a recipe for class unrest. Second, the great fragrance company Firmenich developed musks (Muscenone, Habanolide) that fortuitously possessed a soapy, snowy sparkle reminiscent of aldehydes. All of a sudden it became possible for perfume to outlast soap without veering off course. Karen Khoury at Lauder, and Alberto Morillas and Annie Buzantian at Firmenich seized the moment: Pleasures. It caught the mood of women tired of loud eighties fragrances. They just wanted to smell clean, and not just transiently, but all day, broadcasting the spotlessness of their intentions. The message was that nothing had been deliberately added, that the pleasant, white radiance was just squeakiness writ large. Unfortunately, the scrubbed bareness of Pleasures begat a faceless breed that is still with us, but one can hardly blame a pioneer for spawning lesser imitations. LT

2007 sample.

Poison (Dior) *huge tuberose* $

Reviewing Poison is a bit like road-testing an Abrams M1 tank in the evening rush hour. People just seem to get out of your way, and if they don't, you just swivel that turret to remind them you're not kidding. This is the fragrance everybody loves to hate, the beast that defined the eighties, the perfume that cost me a couple of friendships and one good working relationship. It is also unquestionably the best dressed-up, syrupy tuberose in history, and in my opinion it buries Amarige and the first Oscar de la Renta in the "make it a night he'll never forget" category. Every perfume collector has to have this, but please never, ever wear it to dinner. LT

2011: The changes that have meant catastrophe for pre-eighties Dior perfumes have been a boon for the later ones. Poison is still sickly syrupy up close, but its radiance has changed: drier, woodier, more transparent, it brings to mind a pile of freshly sawn planks. A welcome improvement. TS

Pour Monsieur (Chanel) *masculine chypre* $$

Pour Monsieur should by rights be sitting under a triple-glass bell jar next to the meter and the kilogram at the Pavillon de Breteuil as the reference masculine fragrance. Technically, it is a fresh chypre, and embodies to perfection the accord of fresh bergamot, sweet labdanum, and austere oakmoss that defines the genre. But beyond that, it also defines the exact timbre and volume that a classic masculine fragrance should adopt: a warm, relaxed, confident voice, quietly melodious and in which you can hear a smile. Listen to it carefully, and you won't need to read Baltasar Gracián's *The Art of Worldly Wisdom*. LT

2011: By 2007, there were (1) Pour Monsieur, the original, a masterpiece and as close to Coty's original Chypre as you could get, and (2) Pour Monsieur Concentrée, which was an attempt at sweetening and modernizing. Chanel says that they have unified the two fragrances, and all we have now is the Concentrée, which begins with a conservative lavender fougère top note, for men who distrust any fragrance without it, and sidles in the direction of the original over time. TS

Pour un Homme (Caron) *lavender vanilla* $$
My dad wore this. The fifties ads for it used to describe it as "un parfum stimulant et pénétrant," which is hilarious considering the supposedly sedative virtues of lavender claimed by aromatherapy. It is, quite simply, a lovely lavender with a touch of vanilla. Lavender possesses, on either side of its herbaceous core, stray notes that tend toward either the minty or the caramellic, sometimes going so far as to be reminiscent of fenugreek. I prefer minty lavenders, but Pour un Homme shows that you can skillfully blend a caramellic lavender grade with a discreet but warm oriental base without bumping into Jicky, while at the same time retaining an overall freshness which inexplicably lasts for hours. Probably the best lavender perfume around. LT

Private Collection (Estée Lauder) *floral chypre* $
Even snobs who turn up their noses at any perfume originating outside continental Europe must give this classic from 1973 its due. It smells to me like a bridge between the French tradition of rich floral chypres and Lauder's own very American soap-powder-bright White Linen. Private Collection was supposedly solely Lauder's personal fragrance until admiring friends convinced her

to sell it. If true, it's proof the lady had good taste: it manages to offset exactly an intensely powdery, rich, sweet, floral bouquet with a handsome, dry, woody style, which reminds me of my rule for dresses, such that the more frou-frou the print, the less frou-frou the cut should be. Thus you get your girliness and you get to be a grown-up too. Beautiful, sunny, and confident, with both radiance and tenacity, this fragrance sits easily next to the big French classics on the shelf. If you've never tried a Lauder perfume, this is a good place to start. T S

2007 sample.

Promesse de l'Aube (Parfums MDCI) *peach rose* $$$$
I've said it before and am happy to repeat it: there is nothing quite as good as a good chypre. Francis Kurkdjian, given what feels like an unlimited formula budget, has done an exceptional job in a completely classical manner. The tune of this fragrance (the name translates as Dawn Promise, after Romain Gary's autobiographical novel) may not be hugely original, but the orchestration will bring tears to your eyes. Everything is right: the proportions, from solar top note to deep drydown; the weight, solid but not heavy; the sweep, majestic and caressing. This is an homage to the fifties, done in the lithe, modern, apricot-fuzz manner of 31 Rue Cambon, which it predates by several years. Superb. L T

2011: A new sample smells not of a sunny duet between orange peel and rose, more of a modern vanilla-wood drone as in Dune. But Parfums MDCI indicates there might have been a problem with the batch from which the sample was taken, since discarded. If your first spray fails to sing and instead starts mumbling, take it back. T S

Rive Gauche (Yves Saint Laurent) *reference rose* $

Probably the best floral aldehydic of all time, Rive Gauche was composed in 1969 by Jacques Polge of Chanel fame and overhauled in 2003 by Daniela Andrier and Jacques Hy at Givaudan. I have no idea why YSL messed with it, and on principle I regret any change or modernization of such a masterpiece. The balance between citrus, rose, and green notes set against a dark resinous background in old RG was wonderful. I have an old (circa 1980) sample and the new one. Comparison is made easier by the fact that the beautiful light-proof metal atomizer is the best possible container for long-term conservation. Old and new diverge right from the start: old RG has a strong tarry note up top that sets the dark, dramatic tone for the whole composition. The heart is very similar in both, and the "form," as Edmond Roudnitska would have said, is unchanged. New RG is lighter, brighter, fruitier. Some of this may be due to instability of the citrus aldehydes over time in the old version. The perfumes converge for about an hour. Old RG has some weird, plasticky off notes in the heart, and the new one doesn't. Thereafter, all the way to the drydown, they follow parallel tracks a small distance from each other, and in my opinion the new one keeps level. If I had to describe the difference in overall effect, I would say old RG was more medicinal, the new one more edible. Both are excellent. Try the new, but if you really prefer the old, it will be available for years to come on eBay and other Web sites. LT

Rush (Gucci) *lactonic chypre* $

Has anyone ever made a more perfect fragrance for a night out? Tom Ford reportedly took about two seconds to say yes to the formula after smelling it, and if anyone seems to take longer, hand him a decongestant. When this milky, woody, peachy-jasmine in its opaque red plastic rectangle arrived in shops, it had a bit of the shock of Dylan going electric: though Rush had the bone structure of the kind, cuddly lactonic florals that had kept nice girls smelling good for decades, it came in a joyful fuzz of hair spray and noise, with a delicious, dissonant Habanita-like base of patchouli-vetiver-vanilla putting a growl in its voice. This is not a fragrance for office, theater, or fine dining; it announces its sloppy good mood for miles about, and woe to anyone in the vicinity who planned on using his sense of smell for anything else. This is large-scale outdoor art. And what's more, though it smells so new, so confident, so reckless, so of-the-moment, Rush manages at every stage to feel cozy and alive, never a cold stranger—this creature may be from outer space, but its blood is warm. TS

2007 sample.

Sarrasins (Serge Lutens) *leather floral* $$$
It is said that the young Belgian composer Guillaume Lekeu fainted upon hearing for the first time the fourth chord of Wagner's *Tristan* and had to be carried away on a stretcher. Were he around today, cured of Wagner and now passionate about fragrance, I would have him sit down before smelling the first few minutes of Sarrasins, and would keep some 4711 handy to revive him if needed. Sarrasins (Saracens) starts with a tremendous blast of properly indolic jasmine. Just when you are finished saying "Very nice" and are beginning to form the thought "Where is this white floral going next?" it briefly modulates to what you think is going to be a

dark, minor-mode leather note and immediately afterward startles you with a refulgent blast of apricots. The leather-apricots accord smells to me like osmanthus, and the duet with jasmine then carries on satisfyingly for hours. I've been a Lutens fan from day one, but of late had trouble liking several fragrances that felt oddly loud, even crude. This one is in a completely different league in both intent and execution, an ambitious, abstract, large, rich, sweeping thing of beauty that smells fantastic on skin, is devoid of any overt orientalism, and could just as well have formed part of the new Chanel collection. A minor word of caution: the fragrance is colored an intense purple and stains paper and fabric almost as wine would. LT

Scent (Theo Fennell) *saffron musk* $$$
Theo Fennell is a British jeweler who sells, among many other essential and desirable things, a solid silver lid for a Marmite tin. His Scent, composed by Christophe Laudamiel, is a wonderful surprise. Pitched as an "old-fashioned" fragrance, it is in fact nothing of the sort, rather a modern masterpiece. It starts with a remarkably creamy-fresh and radiant accord of saffron and musk. Then something strange happens. It turns into a Guerlain Transformer. First a lavender-vanillic note kicks in that makes it sidle up to Mouchoir de Monsieur. An hour later it has morphed into a warm woody-powdery fragrance (say Attrape-Coeurs). Later still an intense woody-ambery accord brings it perilously close to Héritage and therefore to all the Héritages-in-drag current at the moment, like Chance. At this point TS and I were ready to watch it drive off that cliff and fall into nasty-drydown hell. It teetered on the edge for a

while, retreated, and, amazingly, went back after twenty-four hours on the strip to the musky-saffron accord of the start. All the while, it amply satisfied the Guy Robert criterion: "A perfume must smell good." It is hard to say whether Scent is better as a masculine or a feminine. Either way, original, memorable, and technically brilliant. LT

Discontinued. It hardly had a chance. O, manufacturer of little faith! TS

Sécrétions Magnifiques (Etat Libre d'Orange)
nautical floral $$
Stupendous secretions! The Dada name had me drooling. The fragrance is both less and far more than I expected: It is not an animalic (supposedly) raunchy thing that works on the assumption that we collect soiled underwear or frequent the same nightclubs as cats and dogs. It is, however, an elegant fresh floral in the manner of Parfums de Nicolaï's Odalisque, given a demonic twist by a touch of a stupendous bilge note, which, my vibrational nose tells me, can only be a nitrile. I remember years ago mounting an impassioned defense of a forgotten Quest material called Marenil, which smelled just like that: oily, metallic, entirely wrong, and begging to be used intelligently. I'm delighted to see it was possible. LT

2011: Smells exactly the same. For the record, there always should have been a dissenting view from me on this one: one star, absolutely revolting, like a drop of J'Adore on an oyster you know you shouldn't eat. Whatever you do, do not allow any to touch your nose when you smell it off a paper strip. I know Luca is a convincing proselytizer, but trust me. TS

S-eX (S-Perfume) *space leather* $$

Felice Bianchi Anderloni, founder of the legendary coach-building firm Carrozzeria Touring (1926–66), was of the opinion that luxury and chic were to a large extent mutually exclusive. In many of his forties cars, he covered the dash with leather and overlaid it with lucite, thereby achieving a properly modern effect that put most other attempts at automotive elegance to shame. Christophe Laudamiel, it seems to me, shares Anderloni's impatience with the merely plush. S-eX is a leather fragrance in the grand manner of Cuir de Russie: rich, smooth, and suitably soft, only overlaid with a shiny plastic accord that obliterates the retro feel common to most leathers and turns it into the smell of a machine nobody has yet had the good fortune to strap himself into. LT

Shalimar (Guerlain) *reference oriental* $$

I hadn't smelled Shalimar on my hand for years before sitting down to write this, and it was quite a shock to do so. The previous memory had faded to its amber-vanillic drydown, that plush, plum-red velvet whiff that says "evening in Paris" as surely as catching a glimpse of the Eiffel Tower lit up for New Year's. Shalimar reminds me of those weird, garish paint schemes, all bold strokes and vivid colors, used on WWI battleships to make them invisible from a distance. Up close, it is intensely woody-smoky, with huge animalic notes, a sort of Jicky wound up like a seven-day clock. From afar, it is a vanillic amber with merely exceptional reach. Shalimar's effectiveness in the middle distance, like the range of a gun, tells you what sort of damage it is meant to inflict. It is not intended for the man who smells it too soon, arm in arm on the way to the taxi. Neither is it a proper boudoir fragrance, a sort of extended dessert. Instead, its uniquely sweet, penetrating tune is supposed to deftly command attention at a dinner party, not so loud that you don't know where it's coming from, not so quiet as to be easily outgunned, above all on excellent terms with the food to come. LT

2011: Shalimar had been getting a bit heavy in recent bottlings, with potent, medicinal vanilla materials threatening to throw off the balance. Damage undone: the most recent version seems to have rebalanced everything, and it's now drier and better than before, nearer Emeraude. TS

Sycomore (Chanel) *smoky vetiver* $$$
The dream team at Chanel seems to delight in applying superior skills to existing ideas they deem worthy of perfecting: Coromandel was a reorchestration of Lutens's Borneo 1834, and of course their Eau de Cologne is a "here's how we do it" object lesson to every perfumer since the 1750s. Sycomore is, in my view, a magisterial gloss on Bertrand Duchaufour's Timbuktu. The latter introduced an Altoids-like idea to perfumery, consisting of a minty-licorice coolness combined with a radiant crackling-wood-fire note. What Polge and Sheldrake seem to have realized is that this accord offered a solution to the age-old problem of vetiver: too little and it gets lost in composition, too much and it always smells the same. Vetiver has both an anisic aspect and a smoky one. Cleverly flank it with Timbuktu's two companions, add a big slug of sandalwood, and vetiver finds itself in worthy company at last. Together they make a strange, very natural accord that shifts from shade to shade of

deepest olive at each sniff. There is a tension, a dark mystery, to Timbuktu, which Sycomore does not try to emulate: it is content with merely being the freshest, most salubrious, yet most satisfyingly rich masculine in years. If putting it on does not make you shiver with pleasure, see a doctor. LT

Le Temps d'une Fête (Parfums de Nicolaï)
green narcissus $

Guy Kawasaki once said that he believed in God because he could see no other reason for the continued existence of Apple Computer, Inc. Now that Apple is out of the woods, I shall redirect my prayers toward Parfums de Nicolaï. Patricia de Nicolaï, owner and perfumer, is one of the unsung greats of the fragrance world, and her superb creations survive in spite of inept marketing, absurd names, and the incapacity of the outfit to settle on a single shade of blue for their packaging or to hire a designer that will finally put their dowdy image out of its misery. This is their latest feminine, and it signals a departure from their ill-advised attempts to make more commercial fragrances. Le Temps d'une Fête is irresistibly lovely. Furthermore, it fills a gap in my heart I didn't know existed. I have always been impressed by the structure of Lancôme's Poême but dismayed by its cheap, angular execution. Conversely, I have always loved Guerlain's Chamade but deplored a slight lack of bone structure, particularly in the latest version. Le Temps d'une Fête marries the two and achieves something close to perfection, rich, radiant, solid, with the unique complexity of expensive narcissus absolute braced by olfactory bookends of green-floral notes and woods. Very classical, and truly wonderful. LT

Timbuktu (L'Artisan Parfumeur) *woody smoky* $$

When I first encountered Timbuktu during a visit to an Artisan Parfumeur shop, I made the mistake of smelling it after revisiting some of my favorites from the firm's distant and more recent past, like Dzing! and Vanilia. By the time I got to Timbuktu, my nose was tired, and I found it nondescript, almost odorless. Nevertheless, I took some home for further inspection. How wrong I was! Timbuktu is probably the first true masterpiece of what, by analogy with nouvelle cuisine, I would call *nouvelle parfumerie.* This school, whose chief exponents are Jean-Claude Elléna and Bertrand Duchaufour, is characterized by complete transparency, an unusually high proportion of high-quality naturals, and what might best be described as the absence of a brass section in the orchestra. This strings-and-winds orchestration gives perfumes that never shout. Timbuktu has a tremendously melodious and affecting start of vetiver, sandalwood, and incense that seems quiet until you realize that, like modern sound systems that can pipe music into every room, one spritz fills a house with an odd, distinctly perceptible, but almost infrared shimmer of woody freshness. No perfume has ever privileged radiance over impact quite to this extent. The central accord in Timbuktu achieves what I thought impossible: a durable dry-woody note without the electric drydown screech of modern synthetics. Bertrand Duchaufour explained to me that part of this effect is due to the use of a rare essential oil from India called cypriol. Having obtained samples from Robertet, I can testify that cypriol, extracted from the sedge *Cyperus scariosus,* is quite something: a smoky note without a trace of oiliness or tar, the smell of crisply burned dry wood on a bonfire. But Duchaufour was being modest: no single raw material ever "made" a fragrance, and he should take full credit for a masterly composition. Timbuktu is the only modern fragrance that replicates, albeit by a completely different route, the bracing, euphoric freshness first bottled in 1888 by Paul Parquet as the defunct but immortal Fougère Royale. LT

Tocade (Rochas) *rose vanilla* $$
It is far too early yet to sum up Maurice Roucel's achievements, since he seems to come up with new wonders regularly, but I would be very surprised if Tocade did not figure among his top three perfumes even twenty years from now. When it came out in 1994, Tocade went against the grain of the two major tendencies at the time, the outrageous and the apologetic, exemplified respectively by Angel and L'Eau d'Issey. Tocade's simple, compact prettiness felt so deceptively familiar that many failed to grasp how original it was. It was a floral oriental among many. It did not use any weird novel molecules. It made no mystery of its intent, which was to have some harmless fun with rose and vanilla, perhaps the two materials most frequently used by perfumers. And yet: if the devil is in the details, so are the angels. Tocade's rose was unlike any other, with the iridescent gleam of nail varnishes that change color depending on viewing angle. The vanilla too was weird, perfectly judged between ice cream, smoke, and candyfloss. Everything, from the juicy top notes to the buttercookie drydown, meshed together perfectly, gracefully, happily, to give a perfume with vivid eyes, a ready laugh, and pretty dancing feet. LT

2007 sample.

Tommy Girl (Tommy Hilfiger) *tea floral* $

No fragrance in recent memory has suffered more from being affordable than Tommy Girl. It's as if it were deemed less desirable for being promiscuous. Despite all the historical evidence to the contrary (Brut, Canoe, Habanita, and the first J-Lo), the world is still crawling with naive snobs who'd rather believe their wallet's loss than their nose's gain. Tommy Girl's origins were explained to me by creator Calice Becker, who was brought up in a Russian household, with a samovar always on the boil and a mother with a passion for strange teas. At Becker's instigation, the legendary chemist Roman Kaiser of Givaudan sampled the air in the Mariage Frères tea store in Paris to figure out what gave it its unique fragrance. From this a tea base was evolved, in which no one showed much interest. The idea waited several years until Elléna's excellent but only remotely tea-like Eau Parfumée au Thé Vert (Bulgari) came out in 1993. Its success made it possible for Becker to submit a tea composition for the Hilfiger brief. She won it, and eleven hundred formulations later the perfume was finalized, in collaboration with a brilliant evaluator who went on to study philosophy. Tea makes excellent sense as a perfumery base, since it can be declined in dozens of ways, as flavored teas will attest: Soochong, Earl Grey, jasmine, and so on. In that respect it could serve as a modern chypre, a mannequin to be dressed at will. Tommy Girl clothed it in a torero's *traje de luces,* a fresh floral accord so exhilaratingly bright that it could be used to set the white point for all future fragrances. Remarkably, late in the project, Hilfiger's PR firm asked Becker to give them some reason to label the fragrance as typically American.

Quest's resident botany expert was called in, and to everyone's surprise found that the composition fell neatly into several blocks, each apparently typical of a native American botanical. So it goes with projects whose sails are filled by the breath of angels. LT

Le Troisième Homme (Caron) *jasmine fougère* $$
For eye candy, both men and women look at women: men are simply not decorative, as everyone knows. Except once in a great while comes a disastrously beautiful boy who turns every head in the street, even if his hair is overgrown, his grubby clothes fit badly, and he's oblivious to the attention as he goes about his ordinary life— he breaks more hearts running out innocently to buy milk than we ordinary mortals manage to bruise in a callous lifetime. Such boys, with their long dark eyelashes, smooth cheeks, and perfect slender bodies, are called "pretty as girls." Le Troisième Homme, named after the Orson Welles film and known for a time as No. 3, is a boy like that, a type of beauty described poorly as androgynous, when what we mean is that it is beautiful before it is anything else, including male or female. I smelled it for the first time on a woman and it caught my heart, the way a stray branch in the woods catches the sleeve of your sweater, and I realized I loved it because of the pitch of my voice when I asked for its name. I've never smelled it on a man and wonder if I ever will: Accidents of nature are forgivable, but how many men can pull off deliberate prettiness? Buy it even if you never put it on. TS

2011: This fragrance had been half girlish jasmine, half the hay-and-musk of daddy's shaving cream. Now it is far closer to the toasty, rum-coffee and lavender of discontinued Yohji Homme. Still great, but not the beautiful androgyne reviewed above. Both would be worth having, though my heart's with the original. TS

Ubar (Amouage) *humongous floral* $$$
I remember years ago seeing an IMAX movie at the Air and Space Museum in DC: it started out with a little grainy black-and-white film of a biplane taking off, and just when you were beginning to wonder why you'd shelled out twenty bucks, the screen turned to color, widened to a huge hollow sphere, and you were flying above a forest in turning-leaf colors aboard a Pitts S2 painted in shiny red and white. Even the sound was gorgeous. Everyone went "aah" and I shed forty years in ten milliseconds. After smelling several dozen pigeon-toed, rickety modern fragrances designed by depressive accountants, encountering Ubar was a similarly joyful experience. This thing is so huge, gleaming, overengineered, and chock-full of counterrotating planetary gears that you feel all you can do is let it tower over you while you walk around it and kick the huge tires. Ubar is technically a floral oriental, but the flowers are XXXL in size and the Orient has been scaled accordingly. If the old Dioressence had an illegitimate child with the first Rush, it would smell like this: a huge purple and romantic rose in the manner of the lamented Nombre Noir; a ton of creamy lactones; a whale's worth of animalic amber. Ubar joins the small club of nuclear-tipped fragrances: Poison, Giorgio, Angel, Amarige. Use it carefully, for once you spray it on there's no going back. LT

Unifaith (Elternhaus) *woody floral* $$$$
Sold encased in a two-part heavy concrete block, this fragrance is, despite the overwhelming artiness, one of

perfumer Marc Buxton's finest works (he recommended I smell it). It is likely the high-water mark of that beautiful style of perfumery Buxton and Bertrand Duchaufour invented independently, the transparent woody floral. Their best creations, from Comme des Garçons to Timbuktu, provide a unique frisson, at once archaic and sci-fi, that brings to mind Le Corbusier's wonderful description of Gaudí's unfinished cathedral as "a ruin of the future." Whereas Buxton's previous fragrances often had a steely sheen about them, Unifaith's admission of floral gentleness into his usual woody severity is affecting as never before. A masterpiece. LT

2011: Beginning life as an art project, this fragrance was listed on its Web site in a font that seemed to say, "Unfaith," and was decorated with a second enormous name, MoslBuddJewChristHinDao, which we took for its primary name in *Perfumes: The A–Z Guide*. We have restored its more cheerful universalist name here. TS

Vanilia (L'Artisan Parfumeur) *candyfloss vanilla* $$$
There's Bad Vulgar (Louis Vuitton handbags, wood veneer in a brand-new car), there's Good Vulgar (flames painted on aircraft engine cowls, John Barry's James Bond theme), and then there's Great Vulgar: Vanilia. Jean-François Laporte was, as always, far ahead of his time in 1978 when he grabbed the wrist of whoever was weighing out the candyfloss (ethylmaltol) in his new vanillic amber and forced in ten times more than anyone had ever dared. In fact, thirty years later nobody has caught up with the unfettered, hilarious, boisterous beauty of Vanilia. It's as if Shalimar met Andy Warhol and came out far trashier and happier. This perfume is so totally devoid of chic it has become the reference hol-

iday from propriety and convention, and by association the purest exemplar of summer fragrance. Enjoy it with a banana float, a sunburn, and really loud music. There will always be time for refinement later. LT

Discontinued. But at last survey, still in stock here and there. TS

Vol de Nuit (Guerlain) *woody oriental* $$$
During the writing of this guide, both authors felt at regular intervals a need to recalibrate their olfactory apparatus to obtain both a reliable zero (Creed's Love in White will do fine) and a full-scale quality reading. The latter can be achieved using almost any one of the old Guerlains, but I find Vol de Nuit is best for calibration purposes because it embodies pure excellence in raw materials and, to me, little else, thereby ensuring that my judgment is not clouded by emotional associations. In truth, VdN (Night Flight), released two years after its namesake—Saint-Exupéry's superb 1931 novel about mail flights to South America—is by Guerlain standards a somewhat shapeless perfume, lacking a legible structure. But it gives me the pleasure, the tickle of anticipation, the feeling of unobstructed space and pinpoint clarity I get when I settle into my seat at an orchestral concert and hear the players practicing. Almost all other fragrances, when compared with VdN, sound like they're being played through the sort of radio people hold up to their ear not to miss the ballgame. God bless Guerlain for still doing this stuff. LT

2011: EU regulations have damaged the softness and richness of this fragrance, which are pretty much all it had. The new one still sort of works, but uncomfortably. LT

White Linen (Estée Lauder) *aldehydic floral* $

Say "aldehydes" in a conversation about fragrance and everyone thinks of Chanel: the groundbreaking No. 5 and the even more aldehydic No. 22. If the aldehydic floral of aldehydic florals, White Linen, done in 1978 by the great Sophia Grojsman, doesn't spring to mind, that is an injustice, but perhaps understandable given that White Linen is neither French nor prohibitively expensive. You simply might not see it, the way you might not see your glasses sitting on top of your head. Lauder's personal favorite (according to the company) is a canonical expression of the American ideal of sex appeal: squeaky clean, healthy, depilated and exfoliated, well rested and ready for the day. Its sharp, biting aldehydes are bright and soapy; the soft musks and woods are a richer version of your favorite fabric softener; the roses are complex, green, and a touch peppery; the whole thing is comfortable and well lit, like a warm spot on the floor where the cat sleeps. (The parfum is softer and more floral than the eau.) I think of it as having a maternal, protective aura, and it reminds me of Thomas Pynchon describing the smell of breakfast floating over World War II–era London as "a spell against falling objects." Guys and gals could both wear it when the sun shines. T S

2007 sample.

Yatagan (Caron) *woody oriental* $$

Caron is home to both one of the most reassuring (Pour un Homme) and one of the most disturbing (this one) masculine fragrances of all time. In the lovely Caron corner shop on Avenue Montaigne in Paris, I witnessed more than one customer recoiling at the smell of Yatagan on his hand, while the sales assistant suavely explained that it was "big in the Middle East," as if some sort of perfume heresy had taken hold *in partibus infidelium*. The truth, of course, was that this 1976 creation and its mysterious Levantine fan club were thirty years ahead of their time. Considered as voices, many masculine orientals try very hard to be warm and husky. More Kaa the Snake than Baloo the Bear, Yatagan goes for a uniquely strange, high-pitched, hissing tone, with odd, borderline sweaty-sour notes of caraway and sage up top, and a dry, inky wood structure below. Respect, or possibly neglect, has spared Yatagan the largely disastrous recent reformulation of Caron fragrances. L T

Yohji Homme (Yohji Yamamoto) *licorice fougère* $$
I shall never forget smelling Yohji Homme for the first time. I was on holidays in Corsica in 1998, and a parcel came from Patou (they used to do the Yohjis) containing a long, distinctive bottle. I sprayed it and fell in love with it so comprehensively that I sat at my computer for a couple of hours just smelling my wrist and staring at the wall. My companions berated me for not going out and enjoying the sunshine, but nothing doing: I wanted to understand this fragrance, write about it while the feeling was fresh, and find out urgently who on earth could come up with something so beautiful. Two tendencies in masculine fragrance had been converging for some time, the woody-fresh (Anthracite Homme, Mark Buxton) and the exotically spicy (Egoïste, François Demachy/Jacques Polge). But their rails could not cross until someone figured out a specially shaped piece to make them merge without derailment. The someone was Jean-Michel Duriez, and the V-shaped material belonging to both worlds at once was licorice. When I

finally spoke to him, he explained that he had been carrying the structure around in his head for years and had found the keystone to his accord in Annick Ménardo's brilliant essay on Angel, Lolita Lempicka a year earlier. There are only two or three masculines out there as good as this. We include it in the guide, despite its being discontinued, in the hope that Yohji's new owners will reconsider. It can still be found on the Web. LT

Still discontinued.

THE OSMOTHÈQUE
by Luca Turin

The Osmothèque [www.osmotheque.fr] is *the* perfume museum, that is to say the only place in the world where discontinued fragrances of artistic significance are stored and displayed. It was founded by Jean Kerléo, then house perfumer at Patou, in collaboration with a small group of senior perfumers, including Yuri Gutsatz, Marcel Carles, and Guy Robert. Its aim was to do what museums do, namely to preserve fragments of the past in good condition, away from the hands of vandals and thieves. In perfumery the vandals and thieves are the very firms that produce perfumes, so this was never going to be easy. Consider this: aside from beautiful aircraft, nuclear power stations, food, and wine, perfumery is France's biggest export, yet there is no perfume museum in Paris. Some will object that Fragonard's museums, one of which is in Paris, do exist, but they are museums of fragrance packaging in the broad sense, attached to thriving and tremendously trashy shops.

For a long time, the Osmothèque was, physically speaking, a basement in Versailles beneath the ISIPCA, France's only independent perfumery school. It organized lectures and visits by appointment and had a stand at all perfumery congresses, usually bereft of visitors. The centerpiece of all these manifestations was always a special carrying case containing small bottles bearing names fit to drive perfume lovers to distraction: Le Parfum Idéal, Jasmin de Corse, Voici Pourquoi J'Aimais Rosine, Le Styx, etc. The intensely knowledgeable

Osmothèque emissary would dip strips for you and hand them over, together with glassine envelopes for you to take them home and savor for weeks and months.

If you visited Versailles and they let you down the stairs, it became clear that the small bottles were decanted from bigger, aluminum flasks kept at constant temperature under argon gas, usually a liter or two in size. The task of compounding those fragrances was the job of Jean Kerléo, and it must have required every ounce of his skill, knowledge, tenacity, and connections. I once in a very small way caught a glimpse of how difficult it must be to re-create a long-lost fragrance. To make things easy, let us assume that you have the formula as written down by the perfumer. If the perfume is fifty years old or more, much of the composition will consist of bases, i.e., subperfumes composed by the industry to make life easier for the perfumer. Many of these bases went the way of the dodo when the small firms that made them went bust, so someone has to remember or guess what they were like. Similarly, some of the grades of naturals may be hard to source. All in all, having the formula may turn out to be like having a pristine Etruscan inscription: you can read it aloud, but have no idea what it means.

As in paleography, life is much easier if you have a bilingual text, i.e., a decently conserved sample to guide the nose and an annotated gas chromatogram of said sample with the molecular mass of each peak identified. There are people, and I have no end of respect for them, who can look at such documents for hours, group the peaks into meaningful patterns, and infer which naturals, which synthetics, sometimes which exact grade of both were used in the composition. At this point the reverse engineering gets in forward gear, and a perfumer can assemble something closely resembling the lost original. All this Kerléo and his able volunteer assistants did to save from oblivion the perfumery equivalents of classical music masterpieces. Jean Kerléo deserves an equestrian statue outside Sephora on the Champs-Elysées.

While the Osmothèque was busy underground preserving the past, the industry, in full daylight, was hard at work traducing it. Reformulation after reformulation, one spurious EU scare at a time, the brands, IFRA, and aromachemical firms collaborated in the wholesale destruction of an enormous artistic capital. Bach and Mozart were wiped out, replaced by Jacques Loussier and Waldo de los Rios complete with drum track. Don't get me wrong: I love both Ray Conniff and Brahms, it's just that I don't mix them. At this point the Osmothèque's refrigerators house not only extinct marvels like Schiaparelli and Rosine, but recent, rapidly cooling stiffs, with labels around their big toes, such as prehypochondria Eau Sauvage, Mitsouko, L'Heure Bleue, etc.

In recent years the rise in interest in nonmainstream perfumery caused by the Web, with its bloggers, boards, and eBay, has been extraordinary and gratifying. There appear to be thousands of people out there interested in the history of fragrance, not merely as an intellectual pursuit but also as a collecting hobby and as pure pleasure. The Osmothèque has as a result become more prominent and more active, as its Web site will attest. It has published books and newsletters of the highest scholarly quality. They are full of accurate information, a rare commodity in the field of fragrance. The Osmothèque is now directed by one of the finest perfumers at work today, Patricia de Nicolaï, who both as owner of a small independent fragrance house *and* member of the Guerlain family has quality in her bones. One of the first things the Osmothèque has done under her stewardship is open a branch in New York City. This presages great things to come, a long way from a dimly lit basement in Versailles.

What, in my opinion, should the Osmothèque be doing? First, at a time when classic fragrances are being destroyed by the dozen, at least keep a stock of the classics and exhibit them as often as possible. Showing the real thing fearlessly will help people realize that they have been paying serious money for fragrance no better than soap-on-a-rope. Second, what the Osmothèque needs is revenue. Ideally some rich enlightened person will one day give them cash to open a venue in central Paris. But in the meantime they should sell their reconstructed fragrances in the museum shop and on the Web, numbered 1 to 400 with no reference to the original name, compounded according to the proper formula. The afición will know its own. Label each bottle with a skull and crossbones and the warning "Do not put on skin" to avoid IFRA trouble. Maybe if they did this they would shame the brands into reintroducing classic fragrances. I'm not holding my breath, not least because I need to sniff my strip of Iris Gris.

L'Origan (Osmothèque/Coty 1905)
In 1904, an ambitious Corsican began an empire in France: Joseph Marie François Spoturno, aka François Coty. A brilliant perfumer, who in time became also, sadly, a repulsive fascist, Coty founded a company that was the most influential in the history of the art after Paul Parquet's Houbigant laid the groundwork for all modern perfumery at the turn of the last century.

Coty learned his trade at the great Grasse firm Chiris

and launched his career with La Rose Jacqueminot, a rich, fruity, liqueur-like rose, and a big hit. The next year he released both Ambre Antique—a simple oriental sketch of balsams that would not be out of place at a niche firm today—and L'Origan. Of these, L'Origan was his first great invention. No natural flower smells like it, and L'Origan certainly does not smell of pizza. (The name translates as oregano.) Instead, it was, like Fougère Royale before it, a fantasy.

Half of L'Origan is a frivolous, fruity bouquet of orange blossom and carnation with a far greater dose of the singular Concord-grape smell of methyl anthranilate than any natural floral extract ever had. The other half is a sweet, powdery, woody oriental of vanillin and heliotropin with a touch of vetiver and dry herbs. Bridging these two very different sides were ionones, violet-flower materials that themselves have aspects both floral and woody. Together they make a greater impression than either a candied flower or a jar of incense ever could alone. The Osmothèque version, fresh and intense, has a stark beauty that age had softened in the vintage samples I've smelled. It leans on your arm both dry and voluptuous, a young woman with chapped lips, in red satin.

Though L'Origan no longer exists—and before it was discontinued its formula had been badly cheapened—if you had to locate its smell among existing fragrances, it would sit between its immediate successor, L'Heure Bleue, and the much later Oscar de la Renta. The contrast between Coty and Guerlain is evident when L'Heure Bleue and L'Origan are side by side: while L'Heure Bleue dreams up a romantic past for every wearer, L'Origan demands you take stock of the urgent news that she is standing before you, right now. T S

Le Chypre de Coty (Osmothèque/Coty 1917)

As one who has never been particularly fond of symphonic florals, I imagine that those who felt as I do must have thought their day had finally come when Coty's Chypre was launched. Chypre, like so many of Coty's great works, was not just a pretty face, more an entirely different kind of beauty. The best way to describe it is by reference to another great success, Paul Parquet's Parfum Idéal 1900. PI is a queen bee's idea of a fragrance: a thousand flowers diligently culled by lesser beings and mixed together like a chorus of praise to feminine luxury. Chypre is what a lone wasp would wear, all business, straight wings, and stark stripes, settling on your hand and walking around briskly trying to figure out whether to bite, sting, or merely ignore you. Smelling the Osmothèque's pristine Chypre is quite an experience. The angularity of it is still shocking all these years later. Fragrances before Chypre had flesh; Coty invented bones. Those bones have over the decades turned out to be so easy to dress a million ways that the chypre category (loosely defined as Coty's brilliant triad of bergamot-cistus-oakmoss) is probably the most successful fragrance family of all time. Smelling it unadorned is like watching an actress take her makeup off while eyeing you in the mirror, slipping some jeans on, putting her arm in yours, and offering to set out into the night unrecognized, paler, and more plainly beautiful than ever. LT

Emeraude (Osmothèque/Coty 1921)

There is so much comfort in unrepentant sweetness that ambery oriental fragrances often tumble into the honey pot headfirst and die a slow, sticky death. How does one extricate these lazy creatures? By adding the essential elements of surprise and contrast without which a fragrance is only a pleasant drone. Over the years, perfumers have found ways to shake up amber: citrus, which predictably works just as well in food, say lemon juice on baklavas (Shalimar); spices and woods that impart a purifying, liturgical feel to the heavy oriental brocade (Theorema, Fendi); and the After Eights idea, warm chocolate and cool mint, a wonderfully dissonant and, for something so delicious, oddly alarming accord. The latter was the option invented by François Coty when he composed Emeraude in 1921. Three things make Emeraude unique: first, the minty-fresh note does not fade with time and instead accompanies the lavish oriental accord all the way through. Second, and this is where Coty's true genius shines through, the fresh part is kept deliberately simple, almost chemical, as a palate-cleansing foil to the rich background texture. Third, the two halves of the fragrance are so carefully welded together that they form a single deep saturated, transparent hue, not so much an emerald as the name would suggest, more the green starboard light of a ship gliding by in the dark. LT

Iris Gris (Osmothèque/Jacques Fath 1947)
The ability possessed by certain fragrances to briefly turn the most arid mind into a fairy garden, to make us lament the passing of loves and losses we know full well we never had, is a miracle specific to perfumery. Alas! Nostalgia, as Simone Signoret said, is not what it used to be, and poetic perfumes are rare, getting rarer. Though never easy to get hold of, Après l'Ondée was at least available and until recently could be relied upon to elicit silent, inward tears on demand. But the mother of all *fées* was always Iris Gris. It was composed, supposedly in a

tearing hurry, by Vincent Roubert. I have heard him described as lazy by industrious perfumers who knew him, with unconcealed irritation at the fact that the gods entrusted a breezy carrier with their most poignant message. Iris Gris is that impossible thing, a hopeful iris, obtained by overlaying the velvet gloom of top-notch iris root with a pearlescent sheen of fresh, transparent red fruit. Sunset dressed as dawn. LT

SOURCES

The Osmothèque in Versailles, France, is curated today by Patricia de Nicolaï, perfumer of Parfums de Nicolaï (see New York, Odalisque, and Le Temps d'une Fête in this volume) and a scholar and historian of the art of perfumery.

In the United States, the Osmothèque is represented by the Academy of Perfumery & Aromatics, a nonprofit operating out of New York City, with the motto "Sentire, Gustare, Amare." Both the French and American offices of the Osmothèque retain samples of its unique collection of historical and reconstructed fragrances and authorize Osmocurators to present them to the public. See the Web site for a schedule of events: www.osmotheque.fr.

Shopping for perfume on the Internet, thankfully, does not require installing smell-o-rama computer accessories. Many stores sell samples for a few dollars each online. Given how inexplicably difficult it can be to come by a sample in a shop, these can be invaluable, since they give you the chance to try a perfume alone at home without distraction and with a big bar of soap nearby in case we misled you and it was all a terrible mistake.

For major brands like Chanel and Estée Lauder, department stores and stand-alone boutiques may still be the best place to try to buy. The chain Sephora wisely gives samples on request, but selection seems to vary from store to store and visit to visit.

For so-called niche brands, which are made in smaller

batches and have limited distribution, specialty retailers, mostly in big cities, are the way to go. You can either contact the fragrance firm itself or check its Web site to find a retailer or just search online. Some fragrance brands have their own dedicated Web stores and may be able to tell you where to find a tester nearby or even send a sample if you're nowhere near.

Two specialty retailers that have helped us over the years are Lucky Scent in Los Angeles (luckyscent.com) and Aedes de Venustas in New York City (aedes.com).

The department stores in which we have loitered longest, trying the patience of the excellent sales staff as we sprayed everything in the room, were Bergdorf Goodman and Henri Bendel in New York, Harvey Nichols and Harrods in London.

To fill in the gap left by stores that offer no samples or small travel sizes, a cottage industry exists of people who are willing to sell you a bit of perfume decanted by hand out of their own bottles and into some third-party packaging, usually plain glass or plastic lab bottles or sprays. The fragrance industry doesn't like this since it removes their control over packaging and retail and prices, and they're concerned, as everyone is, about fakes and contamination. Yet they've been surprisingly slow to meet the demand for smaller bottles and online sampling. If you're in the USA, can't get a branded sample, and don't mind buying a few milliliters of someone's perfume in a plain bottle, an outfit like The Perfumed Court (theperfumedcourt.com), which does a brisk business in clean, well-labeled decants, may be what you're after.

Finally, if you've really gone nuts for perfume and are interested in learning to recognize perfumery materials—what are these ionones we keep talking about? what does bergamot smell like?—an online outfit called The Perfumer's Apprentice (perfumersapprentice.com) offers Perfumery Education Kits exactly for that purpose. It is one thing for us to tell you that some aspect of orris (iris root extract) smells like boiling pasta; it is another thing for you to smell the spaghetti in it yourself.

GLOSSARY OF MATERIALS
AND TERMS

absolute A solvent-extracted fragrance material, traditionally from more delicate natural substances, such as jasmine, which would be damaged by the high temperatures of steam distillation. When both an absolute and a steam-distilled essential oil are made from the same material, as is the case with rose, they tend to differ greatly due to the lower temperature of the solvent versus the steam. Traditional absolutes are derived by using alcohol to extract the fragrance from what is known as a *concrete*, a semisolid extraction of waxes and other substances as well as fragrance, though modern solvents may allow direct extraction of the absolute.

accord Several notes combined to create an effect; related to the idea of a musical chord.

aldehyde An organic compound that ends in a C=O(H) group. Perfumers use many different aldehydes in their palettes.

aldehydic Characterized by the smell of the straight-chain aliphatic aldehydes C10, C11, and C12, first used prominently in Chanel No. 5.

amber A blend of fragrant resins, such as styrax, benzoin, and cistus labdanum, traditional to the Middle East.

animalic Characterized by bodily smells, or smells most associated with traditional animal materials, such as musk, castoreum, or civet.

balsamic Characterized by sweet-smelling fragrant plant resins, typically balsam of Peru, or tolu balsam.

base A prefabricated building block of fragrance composed of various materials and used as a single material by perfumers, such as the famous peach base Persicol.

chypre A genre of perfume built on a structure made famous by Coty's Chypre from 1917, based on oakmoss, cistus labdanum, and bergamot. Chypres can be further divided into floral chypres, fruity chypres, leather chypres, and so on.

cistus labdanum A resin extracted from the leaves and branches of a flowering shrub known as a rockrose. Sometimes called simply cistus or labdanum, it has a sweet woody smell with smoky or leathery aspects, and is a traditional amber material.

civet Traditional perfumery material obtained from glands of the civet cat, usually cultivated in Ethiopia. It has a powerfully fecal character when pure. Civet has been largely replaced in perfumery by synthetic substitutes.

cologne The oldest extant fragrance genre, dating at least from the 1700s. Traditional eau de cologne is a blend of citrus, florals, herbs, and woods.

damascone Powerful materials with rosy-apple smells, related to the ionones of violets.

dihydromyrcenol Woody-citrus material much used in recent masculines.

drydown The late stage of a fragrance that develops after the top and heart notes subside and before the smell completely fades.

ester Combination of an acid and an alcohol that typically but not always gives a fruity smell.

fine fragrance Fragrance sold as fragrance, and not as the scent of another product.

fougère A mostly masculine genre based on the original

Fougère Royale, an abstract composition of lavender, oakmoss, and the tobacco-and-hay note of coumarin.

functional fragrance Scent for functional products, such as soaps and cosmetics.

galbanum A plant resin used since ancient times in medicines, incenses, and perfumes, notable for its distinctive bitter green smell.

gourmand A subset of orientals that has become more popular in recent years, designed to smell distinctly dessert-like with emphasis on vanilla.

green Smelling of cut grass or leaves.

heart note The middle portion of a fragrance, after the top note subsides but before the drydown, often considered to be the fragrance's true personality.

hedione An aromachemical used to impart a feel of dewy freshness to florals, first used significantly in Eau Sauvage.

IFRA International Fragrance Association, the international self-regulatory body of the fragrance industry.

ionone Type of aromachemical that gives the main smell of violet flowers.

iris An extract of the rhizome of the iris plant. Among the most expensive natural materials in perfumery. Also known as iris butter, orris, or orris butter.

irone Type of aromachemical that gives the main smell character of iris.

ISIPCA Institut Supérieur International du Parfum, de la Cosmetique et de l'Aromatique Alimentaire, the only professional perfumery school outside of private firms.

ketone A molecule containing a $C=O$ group, which often confers a nail polish–remover odor character.

lactonic Characterized by perfumery materials containing cyclic ester structures known as lactones, such as peach lactone and milk lactone, which can give a creamy-fruity smell to fragrances.

leather In perfumery, characterized by bitter-smelling isoquinolines or smoky-smelling rectified birch tar, to replicate the smell of the tanning chemicals used to prepare leather.

musk Traditionally an extract of the pods of the Himalayan musk deer, used both for its smell and for its fixative qualities in perfume, now largely replaced by various cheaper, more reliable synthetics.

niche Type of fragrance firm that produces in limited quantity and sells in few shops.

nitro musk The first generation of synthetic musks, discovered in 1888 by Albert Baur, now restricted or banned due to concerns about photosensitization and neurotoxicity.

note An isolated smell in a fragrance (e.g., a note of jasmine).

oakmoss [also tree moss] Different species of mosses from which are extracted dry, bitter-smelling materials essential to chypre fragrances.

oriental A fragrance genre typified by an emphasis on amber, with the oldest surviving member being Shalimar. The genre may be subdivided into floral orientals, spicy orientals, woody orientals, and gourmand orientals.

phenolic Smelling of phenols, i.e., like tar.

reformulation An adjustment to the composition of a perfume. Reformulations range from minor rebalancing, to account for fluctuations in quality of materials, to major new composition, changing the character of the scent substantially. They may be done for budgetary, aesthetic, regulatory, or other practical reasons, such as issues of supply.

resin Thick, brown, sticky plant extracts such as labdanum or styrax that resemble molasses, used frequently in amber orientals or in chypres for their sweet smells and fixative qualities.

soliflore A fragrance meant to represent a single flower. For example, a rose soliflore is designed to smell solely of rose.

top note The first few minutes of a fragrance, when the materials with the lowest molecular weights and highest volatilities evaporate first.

woody amber A type of synthetic aromachemical now widely used to replace more expensive natural woods and ambergris. Woody ambers smell like very strong versions of rubbing alcohol.

Best feminines
- Angel
- Après l'Ondée
- Black
- Bois de Violette
- Boucheron
- L'Heure Bleue
- Homage
- Mitsouko
- Rive Gauche
- Shalimar

Best masculines
- Azzaro pour Homme
- Derby
- Eau de Guerlain
- Habit Rouge
- Knize Ten
- New York
- Ormonde Men
- Pour Monsieur
- Sycomore
- Timbuktu

Best feminines for men
- Après l'Ondée
- Azurée
- Bandit
- Calandre
- Diorella
- Dzing!
- Jicky
- Mitsouko
- Pleasures
- Tommy Girl

Best masculines for women
- Beyond Paradise Men
- Cool Water
- Dior Homme
- Eau Sauvage
- Knize Ten
- New York
- Pour un Homme
- Timbuktu
- Yatagan
- Yohji Homme

Best florals
- Amouage Gold
- Beyond Paradise
- Chamade
- Fracas
- Joy
- No. 5 parfum
- Odalisque
- Osmanthe Yunnan
- Promesse de l'Aube
- Rive Gauche

Best bang for the buck
- Azurée
- Breath of God
- Cool Water
- Knowing
- Lavender
- New York
- Pour Monsieur
- Tocade
- Tommy Girl
- White Linen

Best big ticket splurges
- Amouage Gold
- Cuir de Russie
- Derby
- Homage
- Invasion Barbare
- Joy parfum
- La Myrrhe
- No. 5 parfum
- Sycomore
- Ubar

Desert Island: LT
- Homage
- Jicky
- Jolie Madame (vintage)
- Lavender
- Nombre Noir (Shiseido, discontinued)
- Paradox (Jacomo)
- Talisman (Balenciaga, discontinued)
- Theorema (Fendi, discontinued)
- Timbuktu
- Vetiver Pour Elle (Guerlain)

Desert Island: TS
- Black
- Chinatown
- Diorissimo (Dior, vintage)
- Fracas
- L'Heure Bleue (Guerlain, vintage)
- Homage
- Knize Ten
- Mitsouko
- Shocking (Schiaparelli, original version, discontinued)
- White Linen

INDEX OF BRANDS

Etat Libre d'Orange
  Sécrétions Magnifiques
Geoffrey Beene
  Grey Flannel
Givenchy
  Givenchy III
  Insensé
Gucci
  Envy
  Rush
Guerlain
  Après l'Ondée
  Chamade
  Derby
  Eau de Guerlain
  Habit Rouge
  L'Heure Bleue
  Insolence eau de
    parfum
  Jicky
  Mitsouko
  Nahéma
  Shalimar
  Vol de Nuit
Hermès
  Osmanthe Yunnan
Histoires de Parfums
  1740
Issay Miyake
  Le Feu d'Issey
Jacques Fath
  Iris Gris
Jean Patou
  Joy parfum
Kenzo
  Ça Sent Beau

Knize
  Knize Ten
Le Labo
  Patchouli 24
Lolita Lempicka
  Lolita Lempicka
LUSH
  Breath of God
Missoni
  Missoni
Montale
  Oud Cuir d'Arabie
Ormonde Jayne
  Ormonde Man
  Ormonde Woman
Paco Rabanne
  Calandre
Parfums MDCI
  Enlèvement au Sérail
  Invasion Barbare
  Promesse de l'Aube
Parfums de Nicolaï
  New York
  Odalisque
  Le Temps d'une Fête
Pascal Morabito
  Or Black
Prescriptives
  Calyx
Robert Piguet
  Bandit
  Fracas
Rochas
  Tocade
Serge Lutens
  Bois de Violette